EVEN AS YOU READ THESE WORDS, YOU ARE GROWING OLDER

Yet the miracle of this extraordinary book is that by the time you finish reading it, you will have many more years of vital, happy, fulfilling life ahead of you than you do at this very moment.

The first thing you will do in this book is take its now-famous Life Expectancy Test that swiftly tells you how long you personally can expect to live even with no changes in your life. You well may find that already you can expect to live to be 100.

From that point on, your chances of reaching 100 and even going to the current limit of 120 increase with every new fascinating piece of information.

Not only that, you will learn how scientists within your lifespan may extend life to 300 years or more.

CAN YOU LIVE TO BE 100?

the book that lets you answer YES!

DR. DIANA WOODRUFF is a university professor and researcher whose investigations into aging have won her nationwide renown.

Other SIGNET Books of Special Interest

CAN YOU LIVE
TO BE
100?

Diana S. Woodruff, Ph.D.

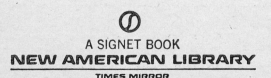

A SIGNET BOOK

NEW AMERICAN LIBRARY

TIMES MIRROR

*To Hyung Woong and his father, Mr. Pak Kyung Koo,
and to my parents, Ruth and Norman Stenen.*

May they live to be 100.

The ideas, procedures, and suggestions contained in this book are
not intended as a substitute for consulting with your physician. All
matters regarding your health require medical supervision.

Library of Congress Catalog Card Number: 77-11997

Acknowledgments

Grateful acknowledgment is made to the following for permission
to reprint or adapt tables, figures, and other materials which are in
copyright or of which they are the publishers:

City of New York (Department of Health), *Family Circle*, Bernard
Geis Associates, Inc., *Geriatrics*, *Journal of Psychosomatic Re-
search*, Alfred A. Knopf, Inc., *Lancet*, Metropolitan Life Insurance
Company, *Preventive Medicine*, Prentice-Hall, Inc., Ronald Press
Company, and Upjohn Company

Full source information for all materials is contained within the
text.

Preface

The early formulation of ideas for this book began in the Spring of 1975 while I was a faculty member at the University of Southern California in the Andrus Gerontology Center. I was asked to be a consultant and panel member for a CBS program entitled, "Will You Live to Be 100?" For their role in getting me involved with that program, I am grateful to Dr. James E. Birren, Director of the Andrus Center, and to Dr. Richard Davis, Publicity Director at the Center.

Mr. Joe Landis, CBS producer of the program, has my admiration for sensing the impact and popularity that a program on personal longevity would have. That program was aired in major cities across the United States and led to invitations for me to lecture on longevity in a number of places including the Governor's Bicentennial Conference on Aging in Honolulu in 1976. Each time I presented the material I was overwhelmed by the interest it generated. I began to see the need for pulling together all of the scientific research on factors influencing longevity and presenting it in a form which would reach all those who wanted to know more about maximizing their chances for a long and rich life. In this regard, I am indebted to Charles Adams, my editor, who put my academic prose into readable form. In addition to the enthusiasm of those to whom I personally presented the material, the press was also interested in the longevity questionnaire. Early forms of the Life Expectancy Test appeared in newspapers and magazines, and when *New West* and *New York* magazines published this material, I was persuaded that I had to write a book to amplify and explain it.

v

The more research I did, the more work I uncovered relating various aspects of heredity, health, social status, and lifestyle to longevity. This led me to enlist the aid of a research assistant, Judith Newman Hornblum, Ph.D., who provided tremendous assistance in tracking down all of the scientific material covered in this book. Thanks to the diligence of Dr. Hornblum, I can say with certainty that there is little research on longevity which we did not sift through in developing this book. Apart from the factors identified in the Life Expectancy Test, few other factors have been conclusively shown to affect human longevity.

Among the material uncovered in the research were a number of life expectancy questionnaires more or less similar to the one presented in Chapter 1. As early as 1920, Dr. Raymond Pearl, one of the major figures in research on human longevity, devised the measure called the TIAL (Total Immediate Ancestral Longevity), a means to estimate life expectancy on the basis of your parents' and grandparents' life spans. More recently, in 1960, Dr. George Gallup published a life expectancy questionnaire based on the habits and lifestyles of 402 people he interviewed who had lived an average of 99 years. Much of Dr. Pearl's and Dr. Gallup's research is included in my questionnaire.

In 1975, stimulated by a number of popular articles which had appeared on aging and longevity, the free-lance writer, Judith Bentley, devised a longevity questionnaire which was published in *Family Health*. It was Ms. Bentley's questionnaire which caught the eye of CBS producer Joe Landis, and it was her questionnaire on which the program "Will You Live to Be 100?" was based. My role in that program was to serve as the gerontologist who validated and explained the relationships on Ms. Bentley's test. The test contained in this book covers some of the same points as the Pearl, Gallup, and Bentley tests, but it is more comprehensive than any of them and is based on more recent scientific data.

There is one final ingredient which made this book a reality. This was the confidence my husband and publisher, Hyung Woong Pak, had in me and in my ability to write a popular book. He was the one who persuaded me to write the book, and he believed in it enough to publish it. Working on this book has caused us to change several of our personal habits in an effort to live a very long time. We both hope that the material will be equally compelling to our readers and that this book will be helpful to many in living a longer and more satisfying life.

D.S.W.
July, 1977

Contents

INTRODUCTION

1.
The Life Expectancy Test: Can <u>You</u> Live to Be 100?

§❧We have the biological capacity to live to be 100. The genetic program for human life extends at least 100 years. There are documented records of people surviving to at least 120 years of age. In fact, biologists currently set the upper limit for the human life at 120 years. So with all these data in our favor, why is it that more than half of us fall short of our potential 120 by nearly 50 years? Why is it that the 1975 census showed only 106,441 Americans 100 years of age and over? The answer is simple, and at the same time extremely complex: we do it to ourselves, and the world around us—with our help—does it to us too. Our lifestyles and our environment are killing us prematurely, abridging our biological right to live to be 100.

"So be it," you say. "Who wants to live to be 100 anyway?" Many people share this attitude. They say that they would rather die quickly and die young than experience the indignities of old age. Given the option of surviving to be

100, they say, "I'd rather not." These attitudes reflect thinking tied to the past rather than to the future, like the ancient Greek myth about the goddess Aurora and her husband Tithonus. Aurora begged Zeus to make her husband immortal, and Zeus granted this wish. However, Aurora forgot to stipulate that Tithonus retain his god-like youthfulness along with his immortality. Tithonus was indeed immortal, but he became old and disabled, and he prayed for the freedom of death.

This notion, that disability and senility are the inevitable accompaniments of old age, persists as a stereotype, even in the face of statistics which demonstrate that 95 percent of the people over 65 live and function in the community. Only 5 percent of the elderly are institutionalized, and less than 1 percent ever become demented. Furthermore, each new generation reaching the age of 65 is increasingly more healthy than the previous one. Negative stereotypes about old age reflect ignorance. Such stereotypes also reflect the unfortunate state of affairs in which there is little respect for old people, and as a result old age is a time of poverty, poor health, and loneliness. The situation is changing, however. In the United States we are gradually coming to realize the significance of population trends in which the proportion of elderly people is increasing. We are also beginning to recognize the value of older people.

President Carter recently called our elderly population America's greatest untapped resource. Steps are being taken by public and private agencies to assure individuals of their right to age in comfort and dignity. Medical advances are making it possible for us to be healthy and vigorous in our 70's and 80's and beyond. Educational advances are creating generations of individuals who will be increasingly more knowledgeable. Improvements in the standard of living and increasing awareness of financial needs after retirement are creating generations of individuals who are better financially prepared for their later years. Mandatory retirement on the basis of age may soon become illegal. Thus, people approaching old age are healthier, better educated, financially better off, and in all ways more able to avoid some of the problems of earlier generations of elderly.

Additionally, there is a growing awareness that we are aging as a society—that the average age of our population is going up. As a result, some of our attitudes about old age seem to be changing. In the last five years more and more sil-ver-haired actors and actresses have appeared on television programs and in commercials. The Pepsi generation is no longer comprised solely of youths. Archie and Edith Bunker have become grandparents. Newspapers carry feature stories on advances in the biology of aging as well as stories on cancer, cardiovascular disease, and how to prevent them. The Grey Panthers and other groups continue to campaign for Senior Power and to draw attention to the rights of older people. Even the federal government represented by the Federal Council on Aging has taken an advocacy role by publishing a Bicentennial Charter for Older Americans (see Appendix). This document was designed as a bill of rights for older people—a relatively revolutionary idea in a country which still persists in worshipping youth.

These early signs of changes in the status and prominence of older individuals in America suggest that as a society we may be entering a new, more mature and human phase. Perhaps the negative stereotypes and attitudes regarding the elderly will be replaced with more realistic and knowledge-able views. These projected changes in the status of the aged, along with the alleviation of many health and financial limitations, puts a whole different perspective on the prospect of growing old. If people knew they could live a full and active life up to the age of 90 to 100, as some do already, they would no longer ask, "Why live to be 100?" They would simply expect it as their right to a complete life. Thus, given the changing social climate and the new prospects for health and financial security in old age, the opportunity to live to be 100 becomes more desirable. The key is to include quality as well as quantity in those extra years, and then the goal becomes something to be actively sought, even prized.

My aim in this book is to keep that goal in mind—to describe some of the factors involved in attaining the goal of 100 years, and to meet the requirement that those 100 years be happy and productive.

CAN *YOU* LIVE TO BE 100?

From the beginning of recorded history we have evidence
that humans speculated on the causes of long life, devised
myths, and invented folk remedies to extend life expectancy.
More recently, we have used scientific methods to determine
and experiment with the causes of long life. While there is
still much research to be done before we can determine accurately all of the factors affecting longevity, a large body of
data has been collected which gives us some clues. Furthermore, this information can be used to evaluate the life expectancy of an individual. Insurance companies have been
doing this for years, and the actuarial tables or life tables
compiled by insurance companies are still one of the best predictors available. For this reason we will use the actuarial
tables as a starting point and begin the estimation of your life
expectancy on this statistical basis. Subsequently, in the life
expectancy test which follows, we will personalize the prediction by taking into account various factors in your background and lifestyle which allow us to tailor the prediction to
you more individually.

Statisticians in insurance companies recognize the fallacy
and risk in attempting to predict individual deaths, and it is
clear that even with the additional, personal information
gathered in this life expectancy questionnaire, totally accurate
prediction is impossible. Thus, the life expectancy test that I
have devised in this chapter should not be seen as a scientific
instrument. Rather, the test should be viewed more as an intellectual exercise than as an absolute form of measurement.
However, it is an exercise which should be taken seriously.
The test points out those aspects of your lifestyle which may
serve to shorten your life, the remainder of the book then
points out the steps you can take to increase your own life
expectancy.

While it is important that you recognize the absolute ac-
curacy limitations of the life expectancy test, it is also important that you recognize how most of the data on which this
test is based were collected, and that these data represent the
most advanced information available to scientists on longevity. (It will become apparent upon reading this book, how-

ever, that these scientists still have a long way to go before they fully understand all the various causes of long life, especially the causes of long life in humans.) Most of the data used are correlational—in other words, correlations or relationships have been found to exist between certain factors and long life. For example, people who live longer tend to have *x*, *y*, and *z* characteristics, while people who live a shorter life tend to have *m*, *p*, and *q* characteristics. Such information does not necessarily mean that factors *x*, *y*, and *z* lead to or cause long life, or that factors *m*, *p*, or *q* cause earlier death—although they may. Correlational studies simply show that certain variable characteristics are related.

It is essential that the reader understand that correlational studies do not provide conclusive evidence about causation. This book will be misunderstood if this idea is not grasped. When a correlational study is undertaken, the investigator measures at least two variables and then statistically calculates the relationship between those variables. It is entirely possible for two variables to be highly correlated and at the same time be totally unrelated. For example, it might be found that the amount of ice cream eaten on a given day was highly correlated with the number of drownings on that day. Does that mean that eating ice cream leads to drowning? No. It simply means that the two phenomena occurred under the same circumstances. In this example, weather is the third variable. On hot days more people eat ice cream and more people also go swimming and drown.

While it is easy to see the absurdity of implying causation on the basis of correlational evidence in the previous example, many people forget or ignore this difficulty with correlational data when variables with some likelihood of being causally related are in fact found to correlate. For example, when high correlations were found between the incidence of lung cancer and the number of cigarettes smoked per day, many were willing to say that smoking caused cancer. Scientists were aware that such an inference was suggested by the data but not proved. Many argued that a third variable (for example, temperament) caused people to smoke and also caused lung cancer. The proof came with experiments showing that animals given large doses of nicotine developed cancer, while animals not given such material did not. This experimental evidence demonstrated a causal relationship.

The obvious reason why it is difficult to establish clear causal relationships in human longevity is that we cannot experiment with human lives. We simply cannot randomly assign some people to one potentially dangerous treatment while assigning another group to a non-treatment condition. The only alternative is to carry out correlational studies of those people who by chance happen to be exposed to the dangerous condition, and we usually do not know if the people in the dangerous group were different to begin with in terms of longevity. Studying such situations provides us with some information, but it does not necessarily tell us the cause.

The correlation between education and longevity is a good example. Data show that people with more education, live longer than people with only a few years' schooling. Is giving a person only a few years' schooling a dangerous treatment? Probably not. The education itself, or lack of it, does not cause an earlier death. The people who were unable to spend a number of years in school are, on the average, poorer, they receive less adequate health care, their nutrition may be inadequate, and they may even have dropped out of school because of poor health. In other words, those who get less education are different in a number of ways from those who get a great deal of education. Education does not cause long life, but length of education is related to variables which are causally involved in longevity.

There are a number of variables which are correlated with long life which are hard to explain at the present time. For example, abstaining from alcoholic beverages is associated with a shorter life expectancy than is moderate drinking. Many find it hard to believe, but those people who refuse to drink alcoholic beverages live an average of several years less than moderate drinkers. This is true even though we know that *heavy* drinking shortens the life span and that excessive consumption of alcohol has adverse physiological effects. It is conceivable that these correlational relationships occur not because refusing to drink affects longevity, but because there is some other quality apart from abstaining from alcohol which characterizes teetotalers and which shortens their life expectancy.

Throughout this book it will be reiterated that the causes of many of the relationships discussed are not clear. It is essential that the reader keep this fact in mind and not make too literal an interpretation of the statistics. On the basis of the data we have currently, it would be unwarranted for a teetotaler to begin drinking in the hope that it would affect life expectancy. It is equally unrealistic to return to school simply because more years of education is associated with longer life. There are, of course, a number of reasons to return to school throughout life, and the fulfillment and purpose which can be gained through learning may indeed lead to a longer, more meaningful life. However, the additional years of school *per se* do not increase life epectancy.

In addition to the lack of information in many cases as to why certain variables are correlated with longevity, it is impossible to know at the present time how the various factors interact. The model used for the present test is additive. In other words, the effect of each of the 32 factors discussed in the life expectancy test is added. There is reason to believe, however, that at least some of the factors may combine or interact to extend or shorten life expectancy in a multiplicative way.

Recent research on the effects of birth control pills and smoking on life expectancy in women provides an example. Smoking and the use of birth control pills both individually increase a woman's (particularly an older woman's) chances of having cardiovascular problems. When combined—by women who both smoke and take birth control pills—the risk of death due to heart disease is greatly increased, much more so, in fact, than the test results indicate when you add together the smoking and birth control pill risks. The two risk factors interact and magnify the effect of one another. There is evidence that the combined effects of smoking and obesity also have a synergistic relationship, further increasing one's risk of premature death. Such synergistic effects are not taken into account in the present test because we simply do not have much information about how risk factors (*or* beneficial factors, for that matter) interact and combine to determine life expectancy. The reader should keep in mind that if he or she identifies a number of risk factors in his/her background and lifestyle, these factors most probably interact to reduce the number of remaining years to an even greater extent than estimated on this test.

Given this qualifying information to help you interpret the life expectancy test more accurately, you should now take the test yourself, and determine if your background and current lifestyle are such that you will live to be 100. Following the test are brief explanations for each of the questions; a more detailed discussion of the factors which affect longevity including what you can do to alter those factors in your favor, is presented throughout the rest of the book.

LIFE EXPECTANCY TEST

The following test is an exercise designed to make you more fully aware of the factors contributing to long life. The test has not been validated, and there is no test currently in existence which can tell you with absolute certainty how long you will live. That which is presented here is based on the best scientific evidence available today. While scientists still do not know all of the variables causing long life, they are aware of some of the phenomena that seem to be correlated with longevity. This test is based on those data. Begin by finding your life expectancy from the actuarial table below, which is based on the latest census figures. On the basis of your sex, age, and race you start with this average life expectancy. Then, by keeping a running score based on your personal attributes, you will end up with a personalized life expectancy and an awareness of what you might do to live even longer. After finding your life expectancy on the table, add and subtract years according to how you answer the following questions.

LIFE EXPECTANCY TABLE*.

Age	CAUCASIAN		BLACK		ORIENTAL	
	Male	*Female*	*Male*	*Female*	*Male*	*Female*
10	70.9	78.4	65.8	74.4	72.9	80.4
11	70.9	78.4	65.8	74.4	72.9	80.4
12	70.9	78.4	65.8	74.4	72.9	80.4
13	70.9	78.4	65.9	74.4	72.9	80.4
14	71.0	78.5	65.9	74.4	73.0	80.5
15	71.0	78.5	65.9	74.5	73.0	80.5
16	71.1	78.5	66.0	74.5	73.1	80.5
17	71.1	78.5	66.1	74.5	73.1	80.5
18	71.2	78.6	66.1	74.6	73.2	80.6
19	71.3	78.6	66.2	74.6	73.3	80.6
20	71.4	78.6	66.3	74.7	73.4	80.6
21	71.5	78.7	66.5	74.7	73.5	80.7
22	71.6	78.7	66.6	74.8	73.6	80.7
23	71.7	78.7	66.8	74.8	73.7	80.7
24	71.8	78.8	66.9	74.9	73.8	80.8
25	71.9	78.8	67.1	74.9	73.9	80.8
26	71.9	78.8	67.3	75.0	73.9	80.8
27	72.0	78.9	67.4	75.1	74.0	80.9
28	72.1	78.9	67.6	75.1	74.1	80.9
29	72.2	78.9	67.8	75.2	74.2	80.9
30	72.2	79.0	68.0	75.3	74.2	81.0
31	72.3	79.0	68.1	75.4	74.3	81.0
32	72.4	79.0	68.3	75.4	74.4	81.0
33	72.4	79.1	68.5	75.5	74.4	81.1
34	72.5	79.1	68.6	75.6	74.5	81.1
35	72.6	79.2	68.8	75.7	74.6	81.2
36	72.6	79.2	69.0	75.8	74.6	81.2
37	72.7	79.3	69.2	75.9	74.7	81.3
38	72.8	79.3	69.4	76.0	74.8	81.3
39	72.9	79.4	69.6	76.1	74.9	81.4

LIFE EXPECTANCY TABLE* (Continued).

	CAUCASIAN		BLACK		ORIENTAL	
Age	Male	Female	Male	Female	Male	Female
40	73.0	79.4	69.8	76.2	75.0	81.4
41	73.1	79.5	70.0	76.4	75.1	81.5
42	73.2	79.6	70.3	76.5	75.2	81.6
43	73.3	79.6	70.5	76.6	75.3	81.6
44	73.4	79.7	70.8	76.8	75.4	81.7
45	73.5	79.8	71.0	77.0	75.5	81.8
46	73.7	79.9	71.3	77.1	75.7	81.9
47	73.8	80.0	71.5	77.3	75.8	82.0
48	74.0	80.1	71.8	77.5	76.0	82.1
49	74.1	80.2	72.1	77.7	76.1	82.2
50	74.3	80.3	72.4	77.9	76.3	82.3
51	74.5	80.5	72.7	78.2	76.5	82.5
52	74.7	80.6	73.1	78.4	76.7	82.6
53	74.9	80.7	73.4	78.6	76.9	82.7
54	75.2	80.9	73.8	78.9	77.2	82.9
55	75.4	81.0	74.2	79.1	77.4	83.0
56	75.7	81.2	74.6	79.4	77.7	83.2
57	75.9	81.4	75.0	79.7	77.9	83.4
58	76.2	81.5	75.4	80.0	78.2	83.5
59	76.5	81.7	75.8	80.3	78.5	83.7
60	76.8	81.9	76.3	80.7	78.8	83.9
61	77.2	82.2	76.8	81.0	79.2	84.2
62	77.5	82.4	77.2	81.4	79.5	84.4
63	77.9	82.6	77.7	81.8	79.9	84.6
64	78.3	82.8	78.2	82.2	80.3	84.8
65	78.7	83.1	78.7	82.5	80.7	85.1
66	79.1	83.3	79.2	82.9	81.1	85.3
67	79.5	83.6	79.7	83.2	81.5	85.6
68	80.0	83.9	80.2	83.5	82.0	85.9
69	80.4	84.1	80.7	83.9	82.4	86.1
70	80.9	84.4	81.3	84.4	82.9	86.4
71	81.4	84.7	81.9	84.9	83.4	86.7
72	81.9	85.1	82.5	85.5	83.9	87.1
73	82.4	85.4	83.2	86.2	84.4	87.4
74	83.0	85.8	84.0	86.8	85.0	87.8
75	83.5	86.2	84.7	87.5	85.5	88.2

LIFE EXPECTANCY TABLE* (Continued).

	CAUCASIAN		BLACK		ORIENTAL	
Age	Male	Female	Male	Female	Male	Female
76	84.1	86.6	85.5	88.2	86.1	88.6
77	84.7	87.1	86.2	88.9	86.7	87.1
78	85.4	87.6	87.0	89.6	87.4	89.6
79	86.0	88.1	87.7	90.3	88.0	90.1
80	86.7	88.6	88.5	91.0	88.7	90.6
81	87.4	89.1	89.3	91.7	89.4	91.1
82	88.1	89.7	90.1	92.4	90.1	91.7
83	88.8	90.3	90.8	93.1	90.8	92.3
84	89.5	90.9	91.5	93.6	91.5	92.9
85	90.2	91.5	92.1	94.1	92.2	93.5

* Life expectancies presented here are based on Life Tables computed by the National Center for Health Statistics for 1975. However, those tables present information for whites and non-whites only. The data for Caucasian men and women are taken directly from those tables, and the columns labeled Black in this table are based on the National Center's category of non-white. This is because 90 percent of the people represented in that non-white category are black. The rest are American Indians (3.3 percent) and Orientals (4.5 percent) and other even smaller groups. Mortality for American Indians is close to that for blacks, and people of Indian ancestry should use the life expectancy for blacks of their same age and sex. However, Orientals in the United States have longer life expectancies than do Caucasians. (This means that life expectancy in the non-white category, which includes life expectancy for American Orientals, slightly overestimates life expectancy for Blacks.) Unfortunately, no life tables are available for American Orientals since they are such a small group in the population. Thus the data given under the heading, "Oriental" are not actuarial data. American Orientals live anywhere from an average of two to four years longer than Caucasians in the United States depending on the source consulted, so the life table presented here was constructed on that basis. To be conservative, two years were added to the life expectancy at each age for male and female Caucasians, and that figure was used for Oriental life expectancy at each age and sex. While this method is not accurate, it is deemed preferable to having Orientals use estimates for non-whites which grossly underestimate their life expectancy.

HEREDITY AND FAMILY

1. *Longevity and grandparents*
   Have any of your grandparents lived to age 80 or beyond? If so, *add one year for each grandparent living beyond that age. Add one-half year for each grandparent surviving beyond the age of 70.*

2. *Longevity of parents*
   If your mother lived beyond the age of 80, *add four years. Add two years* if your father lived beyond 80. You benefit more if your mother lived a long time than if your father did.

3. *Cardiovascular disease of close relatives*
   If any parent, grandparent, sister, or brother died of a heart attack, stroke, or arteriosclerosis before the age of 50, *subtract four years for each incidence.* If any of those close relatives died of the above before the age of 60, *subtract two years for each incidence.*

4. *Other hereditable diseases of close relatives*
   Have any parents, grandparents, sisters, or brothers died before the age of 60 of diabetes mellitus or peptic ulcer? *Subtract three years for each incidence.* If any of these close relatives died before 60 of stomach cancer, *subtract two years.* Women whose close female relatives have died before 60 of breast cancer should also *subtract two years.* Finally, if any close relatives have died before age of 60 of any cause except accidents or homicide, *subtract one year for each incidence.*

5. *Childbearing*
   Women who have never had children are more likely to be in poor health, and they also are at a greater risk for breast cancer. Therefore, if you can't or don't plan to have children, or if you are over 40 and have never had children, *subtract one-half year.* Women who have a large number of children tax their bodies. If you've had over seven children, or plan to, *subtract one year.*

6. *Mother's age at your birth*

Was your mother over the age of 35 or under the age of 18 when you were born? If so, *subtract one year*.

7. *Birth order*

Are you the first born in your family? If so, *add one year*.

8. *Intelligence*

How intelligent are you? Is your intelligence below average, average, above average, or superior? If you feel that your intelligence is superior, that is, if you feel that you are smarter than almost anyone you know, *add two years*.

HEALTH

9. *Weight*

Are you currently overweight? Find your ideal weight on Table A. If you weigh more than the figure on Table A, calculate the percentage by which you are overweight, and *subtract the appropriate number of years shown on Table B*. If you have been overweight at any point in your life, or if your weight has periodically fluctuated by more than ten pounds since high school, *subtract two years*.

10. *Dietary habits*

Do you prefer vegetables, fruits, and simple foods to foods high in fat and sugar, and do you *always* stop eating before you feel really full? If the honest answer to both questions is yes, *add one year*.

11. *Smoking*

How much do you smoke? If you smoke two or more packs of cigarettes a day, *subtract twelve years*. If you smoke between one and two packs a day, *subtract seven years*. If you smoke less than a pack a day, *subtract two years*. If you have quit smoking, congratulations, you subtract no years at all!

TABLE A. Weight, Height, Age Tables
(Ages Twenty-five and Over)

DESIRABLE WEIGHTS FOR MEN			
HEIGHT (IN SHOES, 1-INCH HEELS)		WEIGHT IN POUNDS (IN INDOOR CLOTHING)	
Feet	Inches	Small frame	Medium frame	Large frame
5	2	112–120	118–129	126–141
5	3	115–123	121–133	129–144
5	4	118–126	124–136	132–148
5	5	121–129	127–139	135–152
5	6	124–133	130–143	138–156
5	7	128–137	134–147	142–161
5	8	132–141	138–152	147–166
5	9	136–145	142–156	151–170
5	10	140–150	146–160	155–174
5	11	144–154	150–165	159–179
6	0	148–158	154–170	164–184
6	1	152–162	158–175	168–189
6	2	156–167	162–180	173–194
6	3	160–171	167–185	178–199
6	4	164–175	172–190	182–204

DESIRABLE WEIGHTS FOR WOMEN			
HEIGHT (IN SHOES, 2-INCH HEELS)		WEIGHT IN POUNDS (IN INDOOR CLOTHING)	
Feet	Inches	Small frame	Medium frame	Large frame
4	10	92–98	96–107	104–119
4	11	94–101	98–110	106–122
5	0	96–104	101–113	109–125
5	1	99–107	104–116	112–128
5	2	102–110	107–119	115–131
5	3	105–113	110–122	118–134
5	4	108–116	113–126	121–138
5	5	111–119	116–130	125–142
5	6	114–123	120–135	129–146
5	7	118–127	124–139	133–150
5	8	122–131	128–143	137–154
5	9	126–135	132–147	141–158
5	10	130–140	136–151	145–163
5	11	134–144	140–155	149–168
6	0	138–148	144–159	153–173

SOURCE: Metropolitan Life Insurance Company.

TABLE B. Risk to Life of Being Overweight (in years)

| Age | MARKEDLY OVERWEIGHT (MORE THAN 30%) | | MODERATELY OVERWEIGHT (10–30%) | |
	Men	Women	Men	Women
20	−15.8	−7.2	−13.8	−4.8
25	−10.6	−6.1	−9.6	−4.9
30	−7.9	−5.5	−5.5	−3.6
35	−6.1	−4.9	−4.2	−4.0
40	−5.1	−4.6	−3.3	−3.5
45	−4.3	−5.1	−2.4	−3.8
50	−4.6	−4.1	−2.4	−2.8
55	−5.4	−3.2	−2.0	−2.2

SOURCE: Metropolitan Life Insurance Company.

12. Drinking

If you are a moderate drinker, that is, if you never drink to the point of intoxication and have one or two drinks of whiskey, or half a liter of wine, or up to four glasses of beer per day, *add three years*. If you are a light drinker, that is, you have an occasional drink, but do not drink almost every day, *add one and one-half years*. If you are an abstainer who never uses alcohol in any form, do not add or subtract any years. Finally, if you are a heavy drinker or an alcoholic, *subtract eight years*. (Heavy drinkers are those who drink more than three ounces of whiskey or drink other intoxicating beverages excessively almost every day. They drink to the point of intoxication.)

13. Exercise

How much do you exercise? If you exercise at least three times a week at one of the following: jogging, bike riding, swimming, taking long, brisk walks, dancing, or skating, *add three years*. Just exercising on weekends does not count.

14. Sleep

If you generally fall asleep right away and get six to eight hours of sleep per night, you're average and should neither add nor subtract years. However, if you sleep excessively (ten or more hours per night), or if you sleep very little (five or less hours per night), you probably have problems. *Subtract two years.*

15. *Sexual activity*
If you enjoy regular sexual activity, having intimate sexual relations once or twice a week, *add two years.*

16. *Regular physical examinations*
Do you have an annual physical examination by your physician which includes a breast examination and Pap smear for women, and a proctoscopic examination every other year for men? If so, *add two years.*

17. *Health status*
Are you in poor health? Do you have a chronic health condition (for example, heart disease, high blood pressure, cancer, diabetes, ulcer) or are you frequently ill? If so, *subtract five years.*

EDUCATION AND OCCUPATION

18. *Years of education*
How much education have you had? *Add or subtract the number of years shown on Table C.*

19. *Occupational level*
If you are working, what is the socioeconomic level of your occupation? If you do not work, what is your spouse's occupation? If you are retired, what is your former occupation? If you are a student what is your parent's occupational level? *Add or subtract the number of years shown on Table D.*

TABLE C. Education and Life Expectancy*

Level of education	Years of life
Four or more years of college	+ 3.0
One to three years of college	+ 2.0
Four years of high school	+ 1.0
One to three years of high school	± 0.0
Elementary school (eight years)	− 0.5
Less than eighth grade	− 2.0

* Estimates based on data presented in E. M. Kitagawa and P. M. Hauser, Differential mortality in the United States: A study in socio-economic epidemiology. Cambridge, Mass.: Harvard University Press, 1973 (pp. 12, 18), and in Metropolitan Life Insurance Company, Socio-economic mortality differentials, *Statistical Bulletin*, 1975, 56, 3–5.

TABLE D. Occupation and Life Expectancy*

Occupational level	Years of life
Class I — Professional	+ 1.5
Class II — Technical, administrative, and managerial. Also agricultural workers, as they live longer than for their actual socio-economic level	+ 1.0
Class III — Proprietors, clerical, sales, and skilled workers	± 0.0
Class IV — Semi-skilled workers	− 0.5
Class V — Laborers	− 4.0

* Estimates based on data presented in E. M. Kitagawa and P. M. Hauser, Differential mortality in the United States: A study in socio-economic epidemiology. Cambridge, Mass.: Harvard University Press, 1973 (pp. 12, 18), and in Metropolitan Life Insurance Company, Socio-economic mortality differentials, *Statistical Bulletin*, 1975, 56, 3–5.

20. Family income

If your family income is above average for your education and occupation, *add one year.* If it's below average for your education and occupation, *subtract one year.*

21. Activity on the job

If your job involves a lot of physical activity, *add two years.* On the other hand, if you sit all day on the job, *subtract two years.*

22. *Age and work*

   If you are over the age of 60 and still on the job, *add two years.* If you are over the age of 65 and have not retired, *add three years.*

LIFESTYLE

23. *Rural vs urban dwelling*

   If you live in an urban area and have lived in or near the city for most of your life, *subtract one year.* If you have spent most of your life in a rural area, *add one year.*

24. *Married vs divorced*

   If you are married and living with your spouse, *add one year.*

   A. *Formerly Married Men.* If you are a separated or divorced man living alone, *subtract nine years,* and if you are a widowed man living alone, *subtract seven years.* If as a separated, divorced, or widowed man you live with other people, such as family members, *subtract only half the years given above.* Living with others is beneficial for formerly married men.

   B. *Formerly Married Women.* Women who are separated or divorced should *subtract four years,* and widowed women should *subtract three and a half years.* The loss of a spouse through divorce or death is not as life-shortening to a woman, and she lives about as long whether she lives alone or with family, unless she is the head of the household. Divorced or widowed women who live with family as the head of their household should *subtract only two years for the formerly married status.*

25. *Living status as single*

   If you are a woman who has never married, *subtract one year for each unmarried decade past the age of 25.* If you live with a family or friends as a male single person, you should also *subtract one year for each unmarried decade past the age of 25.* However, if you are a man who has never married and are living alone, *subtract two years for each unmarried decade past the age of 25.*

26. Life changes
Are you always changing things in your life; changing jobs, changing residences, changing friends and/or spouses, changing your appearance? If so, *subtract two years.* Too much change is stressful.

27. Friendship
Do you generally like people and have at least two friends in whom you can confide almost all the details of your life? If so, *add one year.*

28. Aggressive personality
Do you always feel that you are under time pressure? Are you aggressive and sometimes hostile, paying little attention to the feelings of others? *Subtract two to five years depending on how well you fit this description.* The more pressured, aggressive, and hostile you are, the greater your risk for heart disease.

29. Flexible personality
Are you a calm, reasonable, relaxed person? Are you easygoing and adaptable, taking life pretty much as it comes? *Depending upon the degree to which you fit this description, add one to three years.* If you are rigid, dogmatic, and set in your ways, *subtract two years.*

30. Risk-taking personality
Do you take a lot of risks, including driving without seat belts, exceeding the speed limit, and taking any dare that is made? Do you live in a high crime rate neighborhood? If you are vulnerable to accidents and homicide in this way, *subtract two years.* If you use seat belts regularly, drive infrequently, and generally avoid risks and dangerous parts of town, *add one year.*

31. Depressive personality
Have you been depressed, tense, worried, or guilty for more than a period of a year or two? If so, *subtract one*

to three years depending upon how seriously you are affected by these feelings.

32. *Happy personality*

Are you basically happy and content, and have you had a lot of fun in life? If so, *add two years*. People with feelings like this are the ones who live to be 100.

TOTAL

THE LIFE EXPECTANCY TEST—
A BRIEF SYNOPSIS

One of the first things which is notable about the life expectancy test is the information on the life tables. These tables are based on the latest census data and predict life expectancy on the basis of age, sex, and race. You will note that life expectancy at age 10, which is the age at which the chart begins, is greater than the figure we will give as life expectancy at birth (69.4 for Caucasian males, and 77.2 for Caucasian females). The reason that life expectancy increases at older ages is because once you survive certain critical periods, your chances for living longer are greater. For example, infancy is a time when the mortality rate is relatively high. When a baby is alive at the age of 1, he or she has a greater likelihood of surviving longer than a newborn baby. Between the ages of 10 and 25 life expectancy changes very little because fewer people die between these ages. The force of mortality gradually accelerates after that and a greater and greater percentage of the people remaining alive die with each succeeding year, automatically (statistically) increasing the life expectancy of their surviving peers.

Life tables are based on recorded deaths at each age, and the life expectancy given for each age is the number of years you have a 50-50 chance of living. The statistics are computed in such a way that the figure given for life expectancy at your age is the number of years to which 50 percent of the people alive at that age survive. For example, half of the white American women who today are 30 years old will still be alive 49 years from now. Half of the white American women who have already reached the age of 79 today will survive to 88.1 years. Some of the women who are now 88 will make it to 100 years, but there are currently so few people who reach 88 that the government does not even include life expectancy beyond the age of 85 on the charts.

Another thing you will notice on the Life Expectancy Table is the significant difference in life expectancy between the races. Blacks in the United States have a shockingly low life expectancy when compared to the rest of the population. At birth, a black male has a life expectancy almost six years shorter than a white male; the black-white female difference is almost five years. This gap gradually narrows until at the age of 65 the life expectancy for black and white males is equal, and after the age of 65 black men can expect to out-live their white peers, the principal reason being that the percentage of black men surviving to this age is so small that those left are a very select group. If nothing else, these data are dramatic proof of the deleterious consequences of second class status. The data highlight a number of problems which must be erased in the United States if more of us are to reach 100. We must equalize opportunity and access to resources so that all members of our society have a chance to attain their maximal genetic potential for life.

Oriental Americans live longer than their Caucasian counterparts. This is interesting in light of the fact that old age is particularly respected and revered in Oriental culture. Whether the attitudes of these individuals contribute to their longer life expectancy or whether diet or genes are the cause has hardly been investigatd. Studies of the causes of greater longevity in American Orientals may help us to extend life expectancy in all races, but little attention has been given to this minority group.

The biggest and most consistent difference on the life table is the sex difference. Women of all ages and all races live longer than men of the same age and race. A female child born today has an eight-year advantage over her male counterpart. This gap does narrow some in later life, particularly after menopause when women become more at risk for heart disease, but it continues to the oldest entry on the table. This significant difference in longevity between the sexes is an inequity not only for the men who die earlier, but for their wives who survive them. The poorest and loneliest group of old people in the United States are widows. From this perspective, longer life for women can hardly be seen as an advantage. The causes of the sex difference in longevity—both biological and environmental—will be discussed in detail in Chapter 3.

Heredity and Family

The first questions on the life expectancy test involve heredity and family influences on longevity. Many of these questions are related to something over which you have little control. It has been suggested that if you want to live a long time, one of the things to do is to pick long-lived parents and grandparents. Longevity is transmitted through the genes and through the opportunities and environment which your family provides. Grandparents have less of an influence than parents on longevity, and this may result from both genetic and environmental causes. Theoretically, each grandparent contributes only a fourth to your genetic makeup through his or her genetic contribution to your parents, while half of your genes come from each parent. Also, parents are more directly responsible for raising you, and they usually have a more direct influence on your lifestyle, health habits, diet, and outlook on life. The fact that your mother may have the greatest influence in shaping these aspects of your life has been used to explain why maternal life expectancy shows a greater relationship to life expectancy in children than does the life expectancy of the father. There may be biological reasons for this greater maternal-offspring longevity correlation as well. Heredity and family influences on longevity are discussed in detail in Chapter 4.

One thing highlighted in the questions on longevity in parents and grandparents which affects other parts of this test as well is the age of the person taking the test. If you are in your teens or twenties, it is likely that your parents are in still alive, and you therefore cannot add extra years. You are also at a disadvantage because you start with a shorter life expectancy on the actuarial tables. Thus, if you are under 30 and score high on this test, you are really preparing early for a very long life and should congratulate yourself. However, whatever your score, as a young adult, you, of all the individuals taking the test, have an excellent opportunity to alter your life expectancy for the better because you can adopt practices conducive to longevity at an early age which will affect the greatest number of years of your life.

Just as you add years if your parents and grandparents were particularly long-lived, so you subtract years if they died prematurely. You lose the most years if close relatives died prematurely of heart disease or diseases of the arteries. This is because disease of the heart and arteries is the number one killer in the United States—accounting for close to half of the deaths in this country each year—and because these diseases clearly run in families. Although diabetes mellitus and peptic ulcers cause fewer deaths in the United States each year (they rank 7th and 15th, respectively), they are highly heritable and should be protected against if they run in your family. Some cancers, such as stomach and breast cancer, also seem to run in families, although the risk of inheriting them appears to be less than in the case of heart disease, diabetes, or ulcer. Thus, although cancer is the second leading cause of death in the United States, on the test you subtract fewer years for certain cancers shown to be heritable because the hereditary link appears weaker. You have to subtract a year for early deaths in the family caused by anything apart from the diseases mentioned above and homicide and accidents because your lifestyle may expose you to these other causes as well. Also, some investigators have suggested that having parents around until they are at least 60 is a protective factor. Children whose parents die early may not receive optimal care and attention.

Birth order is also correlated with longevity, and the earlier in the family you were born, the greater your life expectancy. It is not clear whether this factor is simply another way of representing the maternal age factor (with later-born children coming when the mother is older and less fit), or whether it is a completely separate factor. It could be social, in that the first born may get more of the attention and resources of the parents. It could also be biological, in that mothers become depleted physiologically after a certain number of children.

While giving birth has some risk to life, modern medicine has made the experience relatively safe, and women who have had children appear to live slightly longer than women who have not. There are several factors involved in this. First, many women are childless not from choice, but from reasons of poor health. Naturally, women in poorer health are less likely to live a long time. Secondly, women who do not have children, whether it is by choice or for health reasons, have a higher incidence of breast cancer. The surge of hormones released during pregnancy and nursing seem to protect the breasts from cancer. On the other hand, numerous pregnancies place great stress on a woman's body, particularly when the pregnancies are spaced close together. Thus, women who have many children experience more stress, and therefore have a shorter life expectancy. Low socioeconomic status puts people at an even greater risk, and since more mothers of large families are in this lower socioeconomic bracket, they are at an even greater disadvantage with regard to life expectancy than mothers of large families in the middle or upper classes.

Intelligence, like so many other traits, runs in families, and very intelligent people live longer than their less bright contemporaries. The advantage may come from being better able to get oneself into an advantaged social position and being more adaptable and smarter at avoiding risks in life, or it may come more directly through the genes. That is, genetic predisposition for higher intelligence may also carry with it a genetic predisposition for greater longevity. This possibility is discussed briefly in Chapter 4, and more extensively in Chapter 10 which deals with education and long life.

While you cannot change your heritage, you can be sensitive to your background and protect yourself from any negative consequences which may come from it. Thus, even if you were not endowed with a brilliant mind, you can behave like an adaptive, intelligent person and extend your life. You can have a family predisposition for heart disease, cancer, diabetes, or ulcers without ever getting these diseases yourself. Furthermore, knowing that these problems run in your family, you can take measures to prevent them. This is what much of this book, and particularly Chapter 5, is about: how to live your life intelligently so as to prevent premature death.

Health

Very few of us will be surprised to find that being overweight shortens our life expectancy. In fact, obesity is one of the best predictors of premature death. If you are heavy, you are putting a strain on all of your organs, particularly your heart and arteries. The reason is that when you are overweight your heart has more body surface through which it must pump blood, and your arteries are clogged with more fat. Heart attack, stroke, high blood pressure, and arteriosclerosis are more common in overweight people, as is diabetes mellitus. Your excess weight also keeps you from being more active, which in turn cuts down on life expectancy in another manner. You are probably not as happy being heavy as you would be as a slim person, and this can affect your desire to live a long time—you simply may not care. Thus, in a number of ways, being overweight shortens life. Furthermore, it is not a good idea to keep changing your weight. If you are overweight, you add years to your life by losing the excess, but you add more years if you keep it off rather than losing the same 20 pounds over and over again. Chapter 6 tells you more about the problems of excess pounds as well as providing suggestions for the best diet for long life. Those who live the longest are just not very concerned about food. They like simple meals and avoid eating in excess.

Smoking is another habit many of us have even in the face of overwhelming evidence that it shortens our life and harms our health. There is no single thing you can do which will add more years to your life than to stop smoking. In the face of all the evidence, no one can reasonably take the position that smoking does not harm health. When people quit, they feel better, their health improves, and their life expectancy goes back almost to normal. Chapter 7 documents the numerous deleterious physiological consequences of smoking and provides some suggestions about how to quit.

Excessive alcoholic consumption is yet another life-shortening habit. Happily, however, moderate drinking is actually associated with longer life. It is not at all clear that the relationship between moderate drinking and longer life is causal. In the final analysis it may turn out that moderate drinkers may be a select group of individuals who have other characteristics such as above average income and occupational levels which combine to lengthen their life. Likewise, people who abstain from alcohol may be those with rigid, unadaptable personalities—such people do not live a long time. Furthermore, the group of abstainers may include former alcoholics who have already damaged their bodies, and it may include those with a genetic predisposition to alcoholism. Such genes may also shorten life. All of the statements to explain the relationships between moderate drinking and abstaining and longevity are hypothetical. The only certain thing at this point is that the relationship exists. If you fall into the category of a moderate or light drinker, you are more fortunate than the individual in the abstainer category, but we do not know exactly why. However, if you are a heavy drinker, it is clear that you are shortening your life. Chapter 8 provides information about the physiological effects of alcohol and the terrible consequences of excessive drinking.

Regular physical activity is something you can do to add years to your life. The activity must be engaged in frequently rather than just on weekends, and it is probably much more beneficial if it is something you enjoy. There are a number of reasons that exercise seems to be related to long life. For one thing, activity affects a number of the organ systems in the body. The effect is particularly beneficial to the cardiovascular system. Your heart pumps blood more efficiently if you exercise regularly, and your circulation is improved. As a result, people who are active have less heart disease. And even if you do have a heart attack, your body is in a better condition to survive it. While activity does not change the level of cholesterol in the blood, it does change the amount of cholesterol laid down in the arteries. This means that your arteries are less clogged if you exercise. Exercise makes your body more adaptive to all kinds of stressors, including accidents and falls. If you work with your reflexes, they will not slow down as much. Your strength will also be affected so that you prevent injuries from accidents such as falls which kill many people late in life. Exercise also helps you to relax. A brisk fifteen-minute walk has been shown to relax muscles as much as a tranquilizer. You can find out more about the benefits of exercise in Chapter 9, along with the type of exercise program you can engage in to improve your health.

Another way of being inactive is to sleep too much. In very large studies of a number of factors related to longevity, it has been found that people who sleep ten or more hours a day die younger. The studies showed that optimal life expectancy occurred in people who stated that they got seven hours of sleep per night. People who slept very little (less than five hours was particularly bad, while less than six showed only a slightly increased risk) also died younger. The reasons for these relationships have not been fully determined. In addition to the inactivity caused by too much sleep, those who sleep a lot may be in poor health or depressed and thus more likely to die younger. The stress of too little sleep may compound the problems of people who are tense and anxious and thus be related to their shorter life expectancy. The studies which proved the relationship between sleep and longevity are discussed in depth in Chapter 9.

The activity and stimulation you get from sexual intimacy appear to extend your life. While there have been no studies demonstrating that humans who engaged in sexual activity lived longer, a few studies of older people have provided suggestive evidence that those who continued to engage in sex lived longer. In animals, experiments have shown that sexual activity is effective in lenghtening life. Indeed, if we were to interpolate the number of years added to human life from the number of months added to rats' lives due to sexual activity, we would gain 12 years from regular sexual activity! However, we chose to have you add only two years in the face of such limited data on humans.

Chapter 3 includes a discussion of the research on sex and longevity, pointing out the benefits to quality as well as quantity of life. Also discussed in that chapter are the differences in life expectancy between males and females and the potential role of hormones in longevity. That male hormones are deleterious to longevity is suggested by the relationship between castration and long life. The life expectancy test includes no item on castration, however, because we felt certain that no male would take advantage of the fact that castration adds many years to life. Animal male castrates live longer as do eunuchs (an average of 13 years longer!). However, regular sexual activity *increases* testosterone level, and sexually active animals live longer. Such puzzles and apparent contradictions have yet to be solved by scientists, many of whom think that the endocrine system (which regulates hormones) carries within it the secret of the human life span.

Preventive medicine is stressed in question 16 regarding annual physical examinations. Many diseases, particularly cancer, are most successfully treated when they are detected early. By visiting your physician each year to check on your health, you are preventing any disease from progressing gradually to the point where it can no longer be cured. Thus, if you practice such preventive measures, you add years to your life.

For anyone who already has heart disease, cancer, hypertension, diabetes, an ulcer, or any other chronic condition, this life expectancy test may be less meaningful. You have already been sensitized to your health, and you are undoubtedly taking some measures to protect yourself from further damage. However, in the presence of these problems, your chances of living to be 100 are not as great as the chances of a person who is without them. Nevertheless, there may be measures you can take apart from those discussed by your physician which will lengthen your life and make it more enjoyable. Pay special attention to the chapters on lifestyle, particularly Chapter 13 on stress and Chapter 14 on personality.

Education and Occupation

The reasons that people with more education live longer are complex. Simply going to school for a greater number of years is not what causes people to live longer. However, education does determine to a great degree what occupation an individual will have. And, of course, occupation affects income. Socioeconomic status is determined by education, occupation, and income. People of higher socioeconomic status live longer because they have more advantages. They can purchase better health care, better housing and food, and they work at jobs which involve much less risk. Their lives may be stressed in far fewer ways than the lives of people of low socioeconomic status. Additionally, people who get more education may be brighter to begin with and have a genetic potential for greater longevity. Success is associated with longer life, and brighter people are more successful. Thus, regardless of education and occupation, if you are successful at what you do (and this is measured in question 20 in terms of above average income for your level of education and occupation), you will live longer. Unsuccessful people often die prematurely. These issues are discussed in Chapters 10 and 11, along with the issue of activity on the job (see also Chapter 9 on exercise) and retirement. Physical and mental activity appear to extend life. Those who are inactive on the job or who are forced into inactivity as a result of retirement seem to live a shorter time than those who can stay active. It is not true, however, that retirement causes death in all people, particularly since many retire because of poor health in the first place. Their poor health precedes rather than results from retirement. On the other hand, forced retirement in healthy individuals who enjoy their jobs is a source of extreme stress, and it may cause some individuals to lose interest in life and die at a younger age.

Lifestyle

Stressors such as pollution and crime are far greater in the city than in the country, and these and other factors contribute to the two-year life expectancy difference between rural and urban dwellers. The pace of life is slower in the country, and it is much easier to be physically active there. More jobs in the country involve physical activities. Nutrition may also be better as country people have easier access to fresh fruits and vegetables and perhaps less access to "junk food."

Just as environmental stresses shorten life, there are also social and psychological stresses which influence health and longevity. These stressors are discussed in Chapter 13. Change is stressful, and although change and adaptation to change are critical to life (and to a high-quality life), too much change affects your health. Presented in Chapter 13 is the "Social Readjustment Rating Scale" devised by Drs. Thomas Homes and Richard Rahe to measure the amount of stressful change you have experienced in the last year. Holmes and Rahe have demonstrated that high scores on this scale, indicating a great deal of change in the preceding year, are associated with a greater amount of serious illness, accidents, and health change of any kind. Chapter 13 should serve to alert you to avoiding too much change, and strategies are also presented for avoiding and controlling excessive stress and change in your life.

One stress clearly documented to shorten life is living alone. Whether you are single or formerly married, if you live alone you have a shorter life expectancy. On the other hand, being married appears to protect you against stress. Close friends also serve as a buttress against stress, and people who like others and who are able to develop intimate personal friendships are happier in old age and seem to live longer. Some of the reasons for these relationships between close personal ties and longevity are discussed in Chapter 13.

Chapter 14 deals with personality and longevity. The most extensive research relating personal behavior patterns to life expectancy has been done in San Francisco by Drs. Meyer Friedman and Ray Rosenman. These physicians developed the concept of the Type A Behavior Pattern which involved a high-pressured, aggressive, hostile personality and a much greater risk for coronary heart disease. Type B individuals, who enjoy life and are much more wrapped up in the quality of their lives than in the material marks of success, live longer and are to be emulated according to Friedman and Rosenman. A questionnaire to help you determine if you are a Type A, along with descriptions of this killing personality pattern and ways to modify it are presented in Chapter 14.

Other dangerous personality traits are tendencies toward risk-taking and depression. Such traits lead people to die in accidents, or through suicide and homicide, the fourth, eleventh, and thirteenth leading causes of death, respectively. Those who are adaptable and easygoing are long-lived, while rigid, dogmatic people die at an earlier than average age.

A final word about happiness. A quality characteristic of most centenarians is happiness. Long-lived people are more likely to say that their lives have been worth living and that they would do it all over again in just about the same way. They have self-respect and self-esteem, they feel needed, and they are happy to be alive. The very special thing about centenarians seems to be the quality, not the quantity, of their lives. Thus, one of the best ways you can succeed in having an extended future is to find happiness in the present.

2.
The March Toward
Living to Be 100

❧Never before in the history of mankind has a society been
so aware of the potential for many of its population to live to
be 100 years old. Never before have so many people lived six
or more decades. To have a large proportion of old people in
a society is a relatively recent phenomenon. While aware—
even in ancient times—of some unique cases of individuals
surviving to reach 100, most people's efforts down through
history have been concentrated solely on surving long enough
to raise or at least bear healthy children, and many were not
even successful in living that long.

In tracing the history of human longevity, it is important
to distinguish between the concepts of *life expectancy* and *life
span*. *Life span* is the extreme upper limit set on human life.
It is the genetic potential of the human species, and factors
that appear to set this upper limit are yet to be discovered.
There is no indication that humans haven't always possessed
the potential to live 120 years. There is evidence, however,
which we will discuss later, that scientists may develop the
potential to change the genetic program for the human life
span. Thus, while accounts of individuals living to be 900 or
more years old are purely legendary, such accounts could become a reality in the future when the key to this genetic up-

per limit is discovered and used to unlock the 120 year human life span.

Life expectancy refers to the average length of life. This is measured by calculating the number of years to which 50 percent of all persons born in a given year survive. Such statistics are computed annually by life insurance companies as well as by governmental agencies, but it is only recently that public records have been kept in such a way that precise life expectancy for the population could be estimated.

LIFE EXPECTANCY THROUGHOUT HISTORY

One of the earliest studies of birth and death rates in populations was undertaken by Graunt and published in 1662. More recently scholars have examined records for earlier periods and made rough estimates of life expectancy. These calculations along with estimates based on more poorly documented pieces of evidence gathered from earlier periods have led to the current picture indicating that human longevity has changed dramatically since prehistoric times. (See Figure 1.) The changes have been in life expectancy, i.e., more people have survived to reach old age. In this way, the average length of life for a given period has been extended over the centuries to the present. The average life expectancy in the United States is now almost 73 years.

Dr. Louis Dublin and his associates reviewed the research on life expectancy throughout history. Studying the characteristics of human bones from the limited number of fossils of prehistoric man which have been found, they estimated that very few prehistoric humans survived even to 40 years. Most met violent deaths at an early age as indicated by fractures in a large proportion of the fossilized skulls. Estimates of average age at death in Greece between 3500 B.C. and 1300 A.D. suggest a gradual improvement in life expectancy from around 18 years in the early periods to 30 years being the average around 400 B.C. Ancient Rome was even a less healthy place to live, with some estimates of life expectancy as low as 20 years. These mortality rates for the highest centers of civilization 2000 years ago are worse than the mortality rate for any country today, but not by much. For example, in a study car-

FIGURE 1. Average Length of Life from Ancient to Modern Times

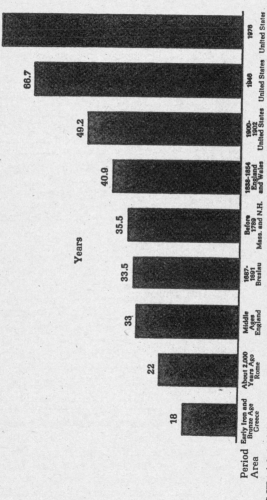

SOURCE: Adapted from L. I. Dublin, A. J. Lotka and M. Spiegelman, *Length of Life: A Study of the Life Table.* Revised Edition Copyright 1949, renewed © 1977 The Ronald Press Company, New York.

ried out for the United Nations, life expectancy in Ethiopia in 1968 was estimated to be 38.5 years.

Studies of life expectancy in the Middle Ages indicate that little improvement had been made over Greek civilization. Estimates for this period range from 30 to 35 years for the average length of life. John Graunt, a haberdasher who lived in England in the mid-17th century, spent his spare time analyzing records of christenings and burials in the city of London. While his data are incomplete, they suggest that life expectancy during that period in England may have been as low as 18 years. More sophisticated analyses undertaken later in the 17th and in the 18th centuries indicated that life expectancy in Western Europe was between 30 and 37 years, and that in selected cities in the United States in this period life expectancy estimates ranged from 25 to 35.5 years. In the 19th century, health conditions improved enough so that about ten years was added to average life expectancy. In the mid-19th century, life expectancy estimates ranged around 40 years, and by the turn of the century, life expectancy in the United States was estimated variously between 47 and 49 years.

It is in the 20th century that we have made the most rapid gains in human life expectancy in the history of mankind. Since the turn of the century we have added twenty-five years to the average life expectancy in the United States so that a baby born today has a 50 percent chance of surviving almost to the age of 73. This tremendous leap in life expectancy has resulted from medical advances, improvements in the standard of living, and improvements in our health care system. Countries in the world which have developed at a pace similar to that of the United States have shown similar advances while underdeveloped countries still have a life expectancy close to that in the United States at the turn of the century. This is shown in Figure 2 which presents life expectancy throughout the world.

Reductions in mortality in the United States since 1900 have paralleled economic progress. The continued development of agricultural and industrial efficiency has led to affluence which to some degree has been used to promote public and personal health. Public funds have been used to build health facilities, to train health care professionals, and to sup-

FIGURE 2. Expectation of Life at Birth, World Regions, 1972 (in Years).

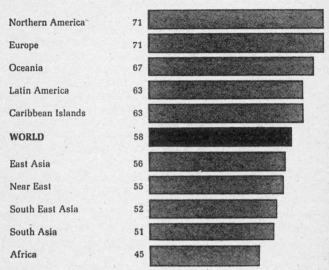

Northern America	71
Europe	71
Oceania	67
Latin America	63
Caribbean Islands	63
WORLD	58
East Asia	56
Near East	55
South East Asia	52
South Asia	51
Africa	45

SOURCE: Estimates from Bureau of the Census, "World Population: 1973, Recent Demographic Estimates for the Countries and Regions of the World," May 1974, pp. 5–11.

port medical research. Increased affluence has also made it possible for individuals to purchase better health care and to avoid malnutrition. Advances in the medical and allied sciences have led to a number of new health goods and services of improved quality. Public health efforts such as the development and application of vaccines, the pasteurization of milk, the chlorination and other protection of water supplies, the improvement of waste disposal, the protection against importation of nonendemic diseases, the improvement of housing (including central heating), the supervision, augmentation, and enrichment of food supplies, and the introduction of air conditioning—all have played a role in making our contemporary life less stressful and more conducive to longevity. Health insurance and welfare have made it possible for a greater proportion of the population to take advantages of health care advances. Additionally, the media has publicized medical advances, and the public has become more health conscious. It will be clear after reading this book that just knowing about factors affecting longevity can extend life expectancy when the individual is willing to take preventive measures to improve health status.

If a single greatest cause for the strides in life expectancy in the last seventy years had to be named, it would have to be the discovery of certain "wonder" drugs. The development of sulfonamides and antibiotics to combat infectious diseases has virtually eliminated diseases which in previous centuries practically wiped out whole populations. The change in mortality resulting from infectious disease is clearly evident in Figure 3 which shows the death rate in New York City for a 150-year period. The tremendous spurts in death rate resulting from epidemics of cholera, yellow fever, and influenza have virtually been eliminated since the advent of sulfa and antibiotic drugs developed in the 30's and 40's. The last major surge in the mortality rate occurred in New York and nationally in 1918 with the influenza epidemic.

Medical and public health advances have had their greatest effect on the early phases of the life span. Infant and childhood mortality rates have been drastically reduced so that more children are surviving to adulthood and old age. While we have not yet conquered the diseases of old age, such as coronary heart disease and cancer, what we have succeeded in doing is conquering acute diseases that affect mortality most in infancy and childhood. Childbirth has also been changed from a risky to a relatively safe event for women, again improving life expectancy. Estimates from the U.S. Public Health Service indicate that if the number one cause of death in the United States, heart disease, could be cured, another six years would be added to our current life expectancy. If all diseases of the heart and arteries, along with strokes were eliminated, eleven years would be added, making life expectancy at birth 84 years. In addition, if a cure for all forms of cancer were found, another five years might be added, making the total 89 years. While these figures are somewhat inflated, since it is highly improbable that total cures for heart disease or cancer will be discovered, scientists have already greatly improved

FIGURE 3. The Conquest of Pestilence in New York City as Shown by the Death Rates from 1804 to 1947.

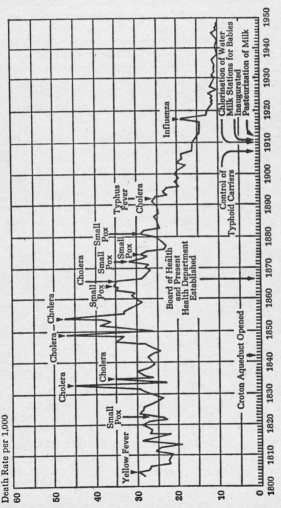

SOURCE: Adapted from "Summary of Vital Statistics, 1947," Department of Health, City of New York.

the chances of survival for people with heart disease or cancer, and this progress suggests that more advances will be made. Thus, it is becoming more and more likely that the average individual can live to the 80's, and the above average individual has an increasing chance to live beyond that. What we will explore in subsequent chapters are the factors which make a person above average with respect to longevity. Before discussing the realities of living to be 100, however, we will explore some of the dreams people had in earlier centuries of living to be 100, and some of the myths they perpetuated as a result of these dreams.

MYTHS AND REMEDIES FOR LONG LIFE

It is ironic that many people in the mid-twentieth century, living at a time when they have a much greater chance having a long life, actually question whether or not they want to live a long time. People of earlier centuries who on the average died at a much younger age had fantasies about long life, and developed myths and folklore to express ideas about longevity. Various rituals and cures to extend life also developed throughout history, again expressing the desires of people in earlier historical periods to realize life expectancies equal to or longer than ours today.

In tracing a history of ideas about the prolongation of life, Dr. G. J. Gruman suggested that myths about longevity have usually been related to one of three themes. The *antediluvian* theme is seen in myths which indicate that people lived much longer in the past. This theme is expressed in the Bible in the book of Genesis in the story of Adam and Eve who were immortal, but who lost their immortality. The life span of many Hebrew patriarchs are also recorded in the Bible, thus perpetrating the antediluvian theme. Adam was said to have lived 930 years, Seth for 912 years, Noah for 950 years, and of course, Methuselah is the best-known longevous individual of all. He was reported to have lived 969 years. It is impossible to document these accounts, and every piece of evidence existing today suggests that the antediluvian theme is only a myth.

The ancient Greeks, who at various points in their history lived from an average of 18 to 30 years, originated the *hy-*

perborean theme which suggests that in some distant place there exists a culture or society whose people enjoy a remarkably long life. In Greek mythology it was suggested that beyond (*hyper*) the north wind (*Boreas*) there lived a fortunate people who were free from all natural ills. These lucky people were never sick, they were able to enjoy leisurely activities and never had to work, and they were never angry or in conflict or combat. This myth is still with us today as we read stories about pockets in the world such as in the Causasus Mountains in the Soviet Union, in the Karakuram Range of the Pakistani part of Kashmir, and in the Ecuadorian Andes where people are reputed to live 160 years or more. Indeed we have even seen the Soviet centenarians on our televisions in advertisements for yogurt. We will have more to say about them in Chapter 12 and throughout the book, but at the present time it is important to note that accurate birth records are not kept in any of the areas where such great longevity is reported. The more literate people become, and the more careful records are kept, the fewer the number of these centenarians are claimed in a population. While the long-lived people of Abkhasia in the U.S.S.R., Hunza in Pakistan, and Vilcabamba in Ecuador are unquestionably very old, it is highly unlikely that they are much over 100 years.

Another ancient theme which is still with us to some extent today is the *rejuvenation* theme. This theme is often expressed by a fountain whose waters are purported to rejuvenate. The best known example of this theme is learned in American history about the exploration and discovery of North America. Juan Ponce de Leon led an expedition to discover the "fountain of youth" and this mission resulted in the exploration of Florida in 1513. Ponce de Leon had heard of this fountain from the Indians, who also believed the myth, and they told the explorer that the fountain would refresh the age and forces of anyone drinking or bathing in it.[1]

Fantasies for rejuvenation and long life seem to be universal, being expressed in the East, in the West, and in the "New World." Dr. Alex Comfort, better-known for his books on sex than for his life-long research in aging, reports that in the 4,000-year-old Smith Papyrus there is an entry, "The beginning of the book for making an old man into a youth . . ."

The remedy was weak, dealing only with baldness and liver spots.

Ancient Chinese practices such as Taichi involved the use of exercises to prolong life. They were developed during Lao Tsu's era (320-350 B.C.), and while such beliefs predate scientific inquiry, research has demonstrated that exercise and activity can indeed extend life expectancy. Many of us take daily doses of vitamin E in the hope that some sort of rejuvenation will take place, and like the ancient Chinese exercises, we do this as much out of wishful thinking as out of scientific evidence that vitamin E makes a difference.

In addition to exercise and special waters and potions as extenders of life, sexual powers have been related to life prolongation. A magnificent monument to the rejuvenation potential of sexual activity is a group of medieval temples at Khajuraho in India. These were built by Chandella kings in the eleventh century, and the temples are famous for their erotic carvings. In the Bible there is the account of attempts to rejuvenate King David in his old age, when he was listless, weak, and cold, by having him sleep with a young, beautiful virgin. Certainly, this is one of the more appealing rejuvenation remedies. Indeed, people who have something interesting in their lives to occupy them probably feel better, and they may even live longer, although, this remedy apparently did not work very well for King David. Ancient Babylonian cuneiform tablets and Chinese pharmacopeoias described aphrodisiacs and preparations with tiger's testes used to achieve sexual vitality and thus youth and longevity. No mention is made, however, of the longevity of those entrusted with the handling of the tigers.

Almost directly in line with this ancient means of extending life was what Dr. Comfort calls the beginning of truly experimental gerontology. On June 1, 1889, at a public lecture, the 73-year-old French physiologist, Charles Brown-Séquard revealed that he had been experimenting on himself by injecting extracts from the testicles of monkeys. He was searching for what we now know as hormones, and he hoped to use them to retard the aging process. His research was ridiculed and he was accused of being senile. Brown-Séquard claimed to feel like a man of 30 as a result of the treatment, but he died five years later at the age of 78.

The French professor's concept was not forgotten, however, and Eugen Steinach attempted to stimulate proliferation of the testicular hormone cells by operating on the testicles. More radical was the Russian surgeon, Dr. S. A. Voronoff, who transplanted the testicles of chimpanzees on to men. With our present knowledge of the immune system, it seems remarkable that the men survived the surgery. Apparently the transplants fell off, and the recipients were left in about the same state as when they came into the operation. While these pioneering attempts seem laughable to us in the 1970's, they represent serious efforts to discover a "cure" for aging. Indeed, in tampering with hormones and the endocrine system which is involved with their production and control, these early scientists were exploring the system currently believed by many gerontolotists to hold the key to aging.

A relatively recent treatment which has received considerable attention from the public—and some attention from scientists as well—is the procane and vitamin therapy, Gerovital. This treatment was developed in Rumania by Dr. Ana Aslan. In 1959 she made claims that her injections of "KH_3" resulted in significant retardation, even reversal, of aging. In her government-supported clinic, the Geriatrics Institute in Bucharest and in its affiliated clinics, Dr. Aslan has treated 45,000 patients. She advises starting regular treatments at the age of 45, but some European physicians converted to her technique claim that 30 is not too early. Twelve to nineteen injections, given one per day, constitute the initial treatment, with tablets given after a rest period of ten days to two weeks. The treatment at the Insitute costs about $60. Hair lotion and face cream made from Gerovital are also available in pharmacies throughout Europe. Among the spectacular results which are claimed are the reduction of invalidism and death among elderly patients, the disappearance of blotches on the skin, the return of hair growth and young hair color, and the improvement of memory and concentration. Such changes make the patient look ten years younger, according to Aslan, and patients also are reported to experience amazing reduction of crippling from arthritis, lowering of blood pressure, and alleviation of depression.

These claims have been somewhat modified of late, but Gerovital is being tested in laboratories in the United States, and it may eventually be marketed here. It may be that Gerovital works as an antidepressant, that it makes people feel better rather than biochemically retarding the aging process. In this light, the Federal Food and Drug Administration has authorized limited research on Gerovital to examine its usefulness in the treatment of depression.

Another treatment which has many strong proponents in the lay (though not the scientific) community is embryonic cell therapy. This treatment was invented in Switzerland in the 1930's by Dr. Paul Niehans, who died at the age of 89. Dr. Niehans got the idea for embryonic cell therapy quite by accident when he treated a patient who had had her parathyroids removed by mistake during an operation to remove her thyroid gland. Niehans injected the patient with fragments of the parathyroid from a freshly killed calf, and she recovered. This led Dr. Niehans to theorize that specific embryonic cells could be used effectively to combat specific diseases. He also speculated that these injections could maintain youthful health and vigor and delay or prevent disease. This cell therapy technique or some offshoot of it is currently used in many "clinics" flourishing from the Black Sea to the Bahamas. Reports on these clinics in *Harper's Bazaar* and *Town and Country* indicate that in Switzerland there are up to 500 practitioners of cell therapy, that there are 200 in France and that in West Germany 25 percent of the physicians use some form of cell therapy in their practice.

The most famous and most expensive of the cell therapy clinics ($2,800 to $3,500 for a week) is Clinique La Prairie in Clarens, Switzerland. This clinic is directed by the successor to Dr. Niehans, Dr. Walter Michel. At Clinique La Prairie the treatment takes one week, and thirty patients can be accommodated at one time. After a thorough medical examination, the patient receives massive doses of fresh cells taken from certain organs and glands of a lamb fetus which was raised in the clinic's special flock of sheep and slaughtered under sterile conditions. Patients are to expect results three and a half months after therapy. They *should* feel revitalized—after the treatment, patients must avoid drugs, hormones, nicotine, concentrated alcohols, sun baths, saunas, diathermy, and hot hair driers.

A number of famous people can be counted among those grateful to Dr. Niehans and his successor Dr. Michel. Among those who have visited Clinique La Prairie are Coco Chanel, the Duke of Windsor, Somerset Maugham, Charles de

Gaulle, King Ibn Saud of Arabia, and Pope Pius XII. Many do report feeling rejuvenated after receiving these treatments. However, since no scientific evidence has ever been gathered which compared treatment of patients with embryonic cells to treatment with a placebo, the claims for embryonic cell therapy are made only by the clinics and the patients who have paid for the therapy.

A modification of this therapy is offered by the Peter Stephan Private Clinic in London. Ernest Stephan introduced cell therapy to England in the 1950's, and his son, Peter Stephan, now runs the clinic using the rejuvenation approach he calls "Body Servicing." The newest treatments are for impotence in males and absence of sexual pleasure in females. Stephan extracts the genetic material and certain enzymes from the cells rather than injecting the whole cell. He claims that this avoids discomfort and allergic reactions. He currently charges around $800 for consultation and rejuvenation treatment.

In discussing this method of treatment. Dr. Ruth Weg of the University of Southern California, suggested that we neither know the effectiveness of Neihans' treatment nor how it works. Dr. Weg argued that the reputed success of the treatment is doubtful because of the body's immunological defenses which break down foreign protein. Perhaps the embryonic cells are broken and used as a source of metabolites and energy, although Weg considers this possibility unlikely. Hence, cell therapy, like so many other attempts throughout history, may be a fraud—working only if and only because the patients believe in it. However, if this belief makes them feel better, then it may do no real harm—unless it steers the patient away from consulting the family physician about health care.

In addition to the many therapies which have been devised to make people physically younger, there is a tremendous demand for cosmetic treatments of various kinds to make people *look* younger. Plastic surgery, and especially the face lift, is an increasingly common means of recapturing a youthful apperance. Men as well as women are now encouraged to use hair products which elimimate all traces of grey. Cosmetics and lotions to preserve youthful apperance are a major industry in the United States, and health spas and gyms designed to maintain youthful looking bodies are proliferating. Thus, on the one hand, we have a history of trying to maintain youthfulness and extend our life span, while on the other hand, we question the goals of living to be 100 and indulge in habits which are literally killing us.

CONTEMPORARY IMPEDIMENTS TO LONG LIFE

While by most measures the United States leads the world in terms of material success, Americans are not among the longest lived peoples of the world. Indeed, Americans do not even rank among the top ten nations in the world in longevity for men. The United States is 16th among the countries in the world for male longevity, and eighth for female longevity. Men survive longer in most Western European countries as well as in Japan, Israel, Iceland, New Zealand, Australia, and Canada. Women in the Scandinavian countries, in the Netherlands, France, Britain, Iceland, and Canada live longer than women in the United States. These comparisons suggest the impact that environmental support systems can have on life expectancy. That government and social conditions can affect life expectancy is dramatized by the vast difference in the average life expectancy between the countries of the world having the longest and shortest life expectancies. In Sweden, life expectancy is 74.7 years. In India it is 46.3 years. Almost thirty years of life differentiates people in these two countries.

Most of the countries with the longest life expectancies have smaller and more homogeneous populations and have generally uniform administration of social and medical support systems. In the United States there is a proportion of the population which does not enjoy the benefits of the majority—including sound nutrition and proper medical care. In third world countries in which adequate health facilities are lacking for most of the population, life expectancy is much lower than in the United States in which a relatively small percentage of the population is deprived. For example, average life expectancy in most African nations does not exceed 50 years. It is clear that a lower standard of living and inadequate environmental support play a significant part in shortening life expectancy. This also means that it is possible to extend the life expectancy by introducing the proper environmental changes.

There are clear steps which could be initiated at federal, state, and local governmental levels which would add years to our lives in the United States. Continuing the attack on poverty, increasing the quality and availability of medical care to people of all income brackets and racial groups, and reducing the homicide, accident, and infant mortality rates would extend average life expectancy a minimum of two years. These steps, coupled with an intensive effort to educate the population about the dangers of over indulgence and the benefits attainable through modifying the high-risk American lifestyle could add years to the life of every American and could result in a country where many more of us would indeed live to be 100.

It seems bizarre that educational and motivational techniques are needed to prevent us from killing ourselves, but that appears to be the case. Although medical science and public health efforts have resulted in greatly extending average life expectancy, the contributions of those professions to longevity were made primarily between 1900 and 1950. We are currently progressing toward our genetic potential for longevity at a much slower rate. This is because many factors which influence longevity cannot be readily controlled by medical science or public health measures. For the most part, these factors must come under the control of the individual. The single greatest life shortening practice in the United States today is cigarette smoking. Obesity is another factor under personal control which greatly influences life expectancy. Stress of various kinds also shortens our lives, and to some extent we are responsible for and we can control the amount of stress to which we allow ourselves to be subjected. Accidents, particularly automobile accidents, are another way in which we shorten our lives, and by simply taking precautions such as fastening our seat belts and observing the 55 mile speed limit, we could increase our chance of survival.

Americans do things in excess. We overconsume and we overwork. Excess calories, cholesterol, nicotine, and alcohol shorten life expectancy in the United States as does excessive competition and striving for success. While medical science continues to develop new means to keep us alive, we nullify such effort by refusing to slow down, relax, and consume less. Alas, the American way of life is killing us at an early age.

But, as America is a country of individuals, there is hope. The individual can and does affect his or her life expectancy, and the purpose of this book is to tell you as an individual how you affect your life expectancy and what you can do to extend it. In Chapter 1 we examined your background and personal habits to estimate your life expectancy on the basis of your present lifestyle. In subsequent chapters we will explore why some factors discussed here and in Chapter 1 are related to life expectancy, and we will discuss what you can do to improve your chances of living to be 100.

HEREDITY

3.
Sex, Sexuality, and Longevity

⁊❧One of the most startling features about the life expectancy tables which you consulted in Chapter 1 is the large sex difference in longevity. A male child born today can expect to live almost eight years less than his female peer. Furthermore, the gap between the sexes in longevity seems to be widening. In 1900 females had only a 2.4 year advantage, but as life expectancy increased over the next 50 years so did the gap between the sexes. By 1964 there was a 6.9-year difference. The most recent statistics indicate that the difference has increased over the last decade to 7.8 years. The most recent predictions of the Census Bureau are that the gap will soon reach a maximum and then level off. There is no evidence that the gap will narrow, however, at least in the next 40 years.

SEX DIFFERENCES IN LONGEVITY—
GENETIC OR ENVIRONMENTAL?

Why does this large sex difference in longevity exist? Do we simply stress males more in industrialized societies in which the gap is greatest? Are there biological explanations based on genetic and hormonal differences? No definitive answers exist yet, but the picture emerging tends to favor biological explanations. Females appear to be the biologically superior sex with regard to longevity.

Evidence to explain sex differences in longevity comes from a wide variety of sources. The starting point favoring a biological explanation is that in most subhuman species females live longer. Since it is difficult to see how the environment favors female animals living in the wild, biologists interpret these data as indicating a genetic and hormonal basis for greater longevity in females.

The most widely accepted biological explanation for sex differences in human longevity involves hormones. The presence of a Y chromosome codes for maleness and causes gonads to form early in fetal development. The gonads produce and secrete androgens or male hormones, and the hormones affect the development of the brain. Indeed, the part of the brain most affected by male hormones is the hypothalamus, that very part of the brain which regulates all further development and which is currently considered by biologists to be the brain center which paces aging. In the absence of a Y chromosome, the fetus develops into a female. Hormonal differences between the sexes affect phenomena such as behavior, metabolism rate, and body structure—secondary sexual characteristics which are likely to affect longevity.

From conception onward throughout the life span, males are more vulnerable. The fact that a much larger number of stillbirths are male than female is further argument that biology rather than environment is involved. It has been estimated that there are 120 males conceived for every 100 females, but many more deaths in the fetal stage are males than females. Thus, at birth the sex ratio is 106 males per 100 females. Boys continue to die in disproportionate numbers to girls throughout childhood and adolescence, with the sex ratio in adolescence being 104 males to 100 females. By the third and fourth decade, male attrition has been great enough to reverse the sex ratio, and during this period of the life span there are only 91 men for every 100 women. The attrition of males accelerates in the fifth and sixth decades leading to a sex ratio of 72 males to 100 females at age 65. By the age of 80, women outnumber men by almost two to one.

One of the emerging problems in a society growing older is the great number of single women in late life. Widowhood is problematic not only because of the loneliness but also it's the most likely cause for poverty in old age. Men are not the only ones penalized by sex differences in longevity. Women who must spend the last ten or more years of their lives alone (because they married men two to five years older and also outlived them by eight years) certainly cannot be viewed as *beneficiaries* of sex differences in longevity.

That greater male vulnerability is at least partially a result of differences in sex hormones is supported by several pieces of evidence. While the sex difference in longevity at birth is almost eight years, if you observe the later years on the actuarial tables in Chapter 1, you will notice that the gap narrows, particularly after midlife. While both men and women have heart attacks—the number one cause of death in the United States—women have them later in life than men. Blood clotting mechanisms are an important factor in heart disease because blood which clots more easily makes the individual more prone to a heart attack. The clotting factor in blood—platelets—are affected by the male hormone—testosterone—making the blood more likely to clot. Experiments have shown that the blood of female animals injected with testosterone clots more easily, while clotting is less in the presence of the female hormone, estrogen. Thus, after menopause, when estrogen levels are low and the relative amount of testosterone in women's blood is greater, they are much more likely to have heart attacks. Men are much more prone to heart attacks in the third and fourth decades of their lives when testosterone output is high.

The most dramatic evidence for a hormonal effect on longevity comes from studies of castration in males. Recent evidence presenetd by Drs. D. Drori and Y. Folman suggests that testosterone may be negatively related to longevity inasmuch as castrated male rats had longer than average life expectancies. The investigators interpreted these results as occurring because of the cancer- and tumor-inducing properties of testosterone in rats. In another experiment, Dr. James Hamilton and Dr. Gordon Mestler, reported that castration prolongs life in some but not all strains or species or animals. To determine the effect in humans, they compared life expectancy of twentieth century enuchs to life expectancy of

matched male and female groups. Castration has been practiced since antiquity, in the West to produce *castrati* singers,
and in the East to provide servants for the members of the
imperial palace and their harems. However, in the twentieth
century only certain cancer patients, psychotics, or mentally
retarded individuals have been castrated. Drs. Hamilton and
Mestler compared life expectancy of 735 intact, mentally retarded men, 883 intact, mentally retarded women, and 297
mentally retarded eunuchs. Not only did the eunuchs outlive
the non-castrated men by 13.5 years, they also outlived the
women by 6.7 years. This is one of the rare instances in
which men outlive women, and Hamilton and Mestler attrib-
uted the effect to testosterone. The younger the men were
when they were castrated (thus, the less they were exposed to
testosterone, particularly if castration occurred before
puberty), the longer they lived. Even men castrated between
the ages of 30-39 lived longer than intact men, however.
Since intact women produce some testosterone, the anatomists
speculated that they, like the intact men, may have died earlier as a result of having higher levels of this male hormone
than did the eunuchs.

Castration is a radical means to achieve longer life in
males. Indeed, most men would not consider it "living" to be
alive in that state. Fortunately, neither rats nor men need to
be castrated in order to have a longer life. Male rats who exercised, or even better, who were given the opportunity to
mate at least once a week, lived even longer than castrated
male rats. The beneficial effects of sexual activity will be discussed later in this chapter.

A fact suggesting a positive effect of estrogen is that
women who have had children tend to live longer. (This is,
they live longer once they survive childbirth.) Since estrogen
production increases dramatically during pregnancy, it has
been suggested that increased estrogen is responsible for the
greater longevity of childbearing women. They are less susceptible to breast cancer and perhaps also to heart disease.

The widespread use of birth control pills (which include
estrogen) on longevity in women is too recent a phenomenon
to appear in actuarial tables. There is suggestive evidence that
birth control pills taken in conjunction with smoking greatly
increased mortality, and estrogen therapy in later life has
been associated in some studies with a higher incidence of

cancer. Thus, it appears that estrogen has negative as well as beneficial effects.

While the biological arguments for sex differences in longevity are compelling, environmentalists may still want to claim that men are stressed more, and that this is what causes their earlier demise—particularly as a result of stress related diseases such as heart disease. It is true that men die in greater numbers as a result of violence and accidents, including occupational accidents. Men also smoke in greater numbers than do women, and they inhale more deeply. In 1972 it was estimated that if all men would quit smoking, the eight year sex difference in longevity could be cut in half. Clearly, this is an environmental hazard which could be reduced. Furthermore, as more women enter occupations—including hazardous occupations—formerly reserved for males, and as more women smoke, we might speculate that sex differences in longevity would be reduced. However, the Census Bureau, in its most recent estimates, does not predict that this will be the case. The Bureau foresees no narrowing of the gap between the sexes for at least the next 40 years. This trend in the face of social changes which are leading to greater stress for women appears to negate the environmentalists' argument even more.

Several studies which provide the most convincing evidence for the powerful effect of biological factors on sex differences in longevity were undertaken by Dr. Francis Madigan under circumstances considered to hold the environment constant for men and women. Social factors in Catholic orders appear to be equated for the sexes. In male and female Catholic teaching orders there are equal health conditions, fairly homogeneous stresses and hazards, and removal from the normal sex roles experienced by individuals who are not cloistered. The nuns consistently showed a longer life expectancy at age 45. This line of research, coupled with the evidence that females of most species in the wild live longer, provides rather impressive evidence that sex differences in longevity result primarily from biological sex differences. Which biological sex differences lead to sex differences in longevity have yet to be clearly determined. The sex hormones, estrogen and testostrone, probably play a role, particularly in heart disease. It is not clear why males are more vulnerable from conception, but again, there is no way to explain this vulnerability at the fetal, neonatal, and early childhood stages other than to simply say it has biological determinants.

However, the growing body of evidence favoring a biological interpretation of sex differences in longevity does not rule out the environment as a potent determinant of life expectancy. Indeed, the extension of life expectancy in the United States and in all industrialized countries has resulted from improving the environment. We are beginning to approach our biological potential for life expectancy by removing or controlling hazards in the environment such as infecton, poor sanitation, and malnutrition. As environmental hazards have been removed, the sex differences in longevity have increased. Unfortunately, as the environment has gotten better for women, some aspects of increasing industrialization have made the environment more dangerous for men. Male deaths due to car accidents, lung cancer, and coronary artery disease have increased since 1900. Generally, however, male life expectancy has increased—but not as much as for women.

The increasing sex differential in longevity has resulted also from social change, even though the current explanations for sex differences in longevity are primarily biological. This is because the underlying biological female superiority was overwhelmed under adverse environmental conditions targeted primarily at the female (particularly through childbirth). As these conditions were improved, the female biological potential could be expressed. This hypothesis would predict that female longevity will continue to rise over male longevity under conditions of continued or increased preferential social treatment.[1]

SEXUAL ACTIVITY AND LONGEVITY

Given that the sex hormones, testosterone and estrogen, are associated with sex differences in longevity, how does sexual activity affect longevity? Unfortunately, the evidence is not as clear as we would like it to be. However, the Abkhasians of the Soviet Union, one of the longest living people in the world, expect to enjoy sex into their 80's and 90's—and they do! Indeed, the story has been reported of the elderly gentleman in Abkhasia who became enraged when his daughter revealed to his prospective bride that he was 108 rather than 95 as he claimed. This was because in Abkhasia a man is considered a man until he is 100. After that it's considered that he is getting old.[2]

Since continuing to be active is one of the primary correlates of longevity, and since maintaining an interest and a role in life is characteristic of people who do live to be 100, it is likely that research in the future will identify continued sexual activity as a correlate of long life. At the present time, however, no conclusive evidence in humans exists. The evidence linking sexual activity to longevity is indirect or based on subhuman species. For example, individuals who are married live longer than those who never marry or who are divorced or widowed. If we assume that those who are not living with a partner have less access to sexual activity, we might ascribe some of the additional time married people live to their continued sexual activity. As we will see in Chapter 13, however, there are a number of factors in addition to sexual activity which contribute to the correlation between marital status and long live.

Indian and Chinese sages advocated sexual activity, believing that it was the means to eternal youth. We noted in the last chapter that many of the remedies for old age and potents for long life involved attempts to return sexual vigor. Western writers, in contrast, have historically taken the position that sexual excess has harmful consequences. At the present time, experts agree that "excess" in sexual activity is not a useful concept due to the tremendous range of individual variation in sexual capacity and interest. Alex Comfort also suggested in 1961, long before writing about the joys of sex, that the Indians and Chinese rather than the monks were right. Regularly mated rats stay in far better health than rats which are prevented from mating. Furthermore, as Comfort wryly remarked—what is true of rats is also true of clergymen. Studies comparing the mortality rates of Anglican and other Protestant clergy who marry to the mortality rates of Roman Catholic clergy who take vows of celibacy indicated that the married clergy live longer than their celibate peers.[3] While these data along with the data comparing life expectancies of married and non-married individuals are undoubtedly confounded with factors apart from sexual activity, it does appear that the virtues of sexual abstinence, at least as they relate to longevity, have been misrepresented by the moralists.

A belief which has remained with us for centuries and which has no basis in fact is that the sexual secretions are the elixir of life and must be conserved if we are not to waste away. Just as men have been urged to conserve their precious juices, so have women been warned of the dangers of an active sex life. Dr. Comfort quotes Lorand who published a book in 1910 entitlted *Old Age Deferred,* as stating, "Even young girls may acquire some of the attributes of old age by such means (as frequent coition). They soon become fat and bloated . . . the cheeks become pendent: There is a marked difference between the muscles of a young maiden and those of a woman who has been leading a life of debauchery. . . ."[4] Authors of the Victorian age were influenced by prevailing social mores to conclude that more than a little sexual activity shortened life expectancy. Authors of the 1970's, living in an era of sexual freedom, favor evidence suggesting that sexual activity leads to greater longevity. Perhaps we, like our predecessors, will be accused of being swept away with the prevailing attitudes of the times by interpreting current evidence to suggest that an active sex life may be associated with longer life. Nevertheless, that is what the indicators today point to.

The most conclusive evidence on the relationship between sexual activity and longevity comes from studies of animals. As early as 1939 research indicated that sexual intercourse increases resistance of male and female rats, mice, and rabbits to toxic substances. In 1969 Drs. Drori and Folman had shown that the mean life span of male rats allowed to mate at least weekly was significantly longer than that of their litter mates who were not allowed access to female rats. But in the group allowed to mate there was a much higher level of circulating testosterone, so why did these rats live longer if high levels of testosterone shorten life expectancy? Drori and Folman's hypothesis was that testosterone is associated with increased activity, and it is the increased activity or exercise that affects longevity. Their 1976 study demonstrated that mating probably increases longevity by increasing voluntary exercise. They compared mated rats to rats unmated but exercised two minutes daily. Also included in this study were groups of rats who were castrated, groups who were underfed, and groups who received no treatment (including no access to female rats). The exercised rats lived as long as the mated rats. In fact, mating appeared to induce even more exercise than engaged in by the exercised group. The lungs of these two groups of rats were affected positively, and both the mated and exercised groups had a reduced incidence of pneumonia. Thus, while circulating testosterone may have deleterious effects, these effects may be balanced by the activity-inducing properties of the hormone. These data imply that the source of the activity, be it sexual or physical exercise, is not important. The activity itself is the significant factor.

It is extremely risky to interpolate the results of animal studies to humans, but there is extensive data from studies on humans indicating that activity is essential to long life. Thus, we might conclude that the Drori and Folman work provides a means for all of us to extend our lives. Those of us with access to a mate can be active sexually. Those of us without a sexual partner can be active physically and benefit our longevity just as our sexually active friends. This prescription of activity, including sexual activity, applies to all points of the life span. Activity in the sixties, seventies, eighties, and beyond is at least as important as it was in earlier periods. Unfortunately, many of us recoil at this thought—particularly the thought of sexual activity late in life. How unfortunate that such a pleasant feature of long life is abandoned by many of us as we age because we feel that it is unnatural.

SEXUAL ACTIVITY OVER THE LIFE SPAN

Formal sanctions for sexual behavior in the United States are only extended by marriage, and while this pattern is not subscribed to by a majority of adolescents, we still discourage sexual activity in childhood and adolescence. In many parts of the country parents spend years teaching children to inhibit sexual responses—presumably to prepare them for the time when they will be expected to make these very responses. Children are taught to respond to sex with anxiety and guilt in early life, expected to perform without anxiety as adults, and then expected to abstain as old people. Sex in Abkhasia, where people are unusually long-lived, is considered a good and pleasurable and guiltless thing. Sexual matters are extremely private, and young people are encouraged to postpone sexual gratification not as a matter of frustration, but as a hopeful expectation of future enjoyment. This is because a continuation of sex life into old age is considered as natural as maintaining a healthy appetite or sound sleep.[5]

Given the values of contemporary American youth, emphasizing the importance of affection and maturity in sex, future generations may be less likely to experience the guilt and anxiety over sexual matters which still expresses itself in the behavior and attitudes of middle-aged and aged generations. In addition to their added enjoyment of life, the life expectancy of these youths may benefit from their outlook.

Sexual activity appears to peak early in life—usually during the first few years of marriage when an interesting and available partner is present. The pioneering work of Dr. Alfred Kinsey was among the first to document that the frequency of intercourse declines fairly steadily with age, and that changes in male patterns of activity pace age changes for both men and women. Both single and married men have fewer orgasms with each successive decade, while the change with age for single women is minimal. A married woman's decline in frequency of orgasm apparently results from age changes in her husband's sexual patterns, since her own sexual capacity continues to increase until mid-life.

While many individuals enjoy an active sex life throughout middle and old age, it is in mid-life that individuals often experience problems with sexuality. Women during this period of their life span are still close to the peak point of their activity, and many women report an increase in sexual interest either because they incorrectly assume that they may soon lose sexual satisfaction with the onset of the menopause or because they are relieved not to have to worry about unwanted pregnancy. Men, however, in middle age and at the peak of their careers, may be less interested in sexual activity and may experience impotence for the first time. The inability to have an erection during intercourse increased in incidence during middle age, and Dr. William Masters and Virginia Johnson reported, after the age of 50 the incidence of sexual inadequacy in men increases dramatically. Normally this occurrence is not due to physiological age changes in the male (who experiences a gradual reduction in testosterone level as he ages, as opposed to a rapid drop of estrogen production at menopause in women). Impotence in middle-aged men appears to be largely caused by social and psychological factors. While certainly there are physical changes occurring in both the male and female which make their sexual responses slower and of less magnitude, these slight and gradual declines can in no way account for the inability to maintain an erection or to achieve orgasm.

Menopause occurs in the middle-aged female as a dramatic sign that her reproductive years are ended. It is probably the symbolic significance of the menopause that has the most impact on women rather than the slight physical discomfort they may experience. Research suggests, however, that even the stressful psychological aspects of menopause are overrated.

The menstrual cycle ends in most women between the ages of 45 and 50 and estrogen and progesterone are no longer produced by the ovaries. Since satisfying sexual activity is not affected by estrogen and progesterone levels, sexual pleasure need not decline after menopause; as mentioned previously, some women experience an increase in sexual interest and activity at this point as they no longer are anxious about pregnancy.

Physical changes such as loss of elasticity of the skin, hot flashes, appearance of facial hair, and changes in the breasts and genitals can be retarded by treatment with estrogen. While many specialists advocate the use of estrogen therapy to retard physical aging in appearance and function, others warn of the danger of increased incidence of cancer. Women and their physicians should be aware of the benefits of estrogen replacement, but they must also be alerted to the potential danger of this treatment. Additional research is underway to more clearly evaluate the relative benefits in light of the increased danger of cancer.

A study of attitudes of women of various ages to menopause was carried out by Dr. Bernice Neugarten at the University of Chicago. Results indicated that half of the middle-class women in the sample had extremely negative attitudes toward this change while the other half had more favorable attitudes. Women beyond the age of 45 (who had presumably experienced menopause) saw more favorable aspects of this period than did younger women. The older women and women who were better educated also saw the change as less stressful, suggesting that the more that is known about menopause, the less problem it creates. Women reported that one of the worst things about menopause was not knowing what to expect. Also rated as negative aspects were the pain and discomfort and the indication that one was getting older. Most felt, however, that menopause had no effect on sexual relations or on physical and mental health.[6]

While most men do not experience anything analogous to menopause, they probably do experience a decrease in reproductive ability late in life when fertile sperm are no longer produced. The rapid decrease in hormone level experienced by women during menopause is responsible for some of the physical symptoms they experience, and Drs. H. J. Ruebsaat and R. Hull have reported similar symptoms in about 10 to 15 percent of men in their mid to late fifties or early sixties. It appears that in this small proportion of men there is a rapid rather than a gradual drop in hormone level, and men who experience this rapid hormone drop suffer physical and sometimes psychological discomfort. Hot flashes, dizziness, and depression have been reported by men with this syndrome. Thus, while there is no male menopause involving both the loss of reproductive capacity and the rapid decline of hormones, some men do experience a rapid drop in hormone level leading them to experience symptoms similar to the symptoms of menopausal women.

SEXUALITY IN OLD AGE

There are a great number of misconceptions about sex in old age held by most laymen and, more tragically, by many physicians as well. Recent emphasis on sex education and on the research of Masters and Johnson which has received widespread coverage by the media may be affecting public awareness of sexual potential in old age. A study of Brandeis students undertaken in the 1950's, in which students were asked to complete the sentence "Sex for old people is . . ." yielded pessimistic answers such as "unimportant," "past," and "negligible."[7] A more recent survey involving students in gerontology classes taught by the author at the University of Southern California and at Temple University led to a more positive picture. Students polled in the 1970's were unanimous in their acknowledgment that sex continues to play an important role in the lives of old people. Students completed the sentence with descriptions such as "O.K., but strange"—"important and gratifying"—"good"—"fun"—"a matter of personal ability, attitude, and opportunity"—"as important as it is for people of all ages for psychological well being. It depends upon individual needs and appetite"—"whatever they want to make it"—"great if they are both capable of doing it"—"not necessarily different than for younger people"—"beneficial"—"groovy but infrequent—"great as long as they can and do still dig it"—"probably more desired than had"—and lastly, the insightful reflection: "still a part of life, and since they are still alive it's cool."

Such data are encouraging not only because they reflect positive attitudes about aging, but because they indicate that future generations of elderly people may have more active sex lives. It appears that the best correlate of sexual activity in old age is patterns of sexual activity in earlier years. Thus, healthy attitudes about sex in old age decrease the probability of a self-fulfilling prophecy. Dr. Rober Butler, Director of the National Institute of Aging has pointed out that those individuals who have a positive attitude about sex and who derive sexual satisfaction in early life will have the best chance to enjoy a rich sex life when they are old.

Masters and Johnson have noted that psychological factors play at least as great a role as hormones in determining the sex drive of older individuals, yet misinformation about sex in the later years often exaggerates fears and misconceptions which sexually incapacitate the aging. There is an amazing amount of misinformation. For example, if intercourse is painful for an older women as a result of slight atrophy in her vulva and vagina, many physicians are apt to say, "What do you expect at your age?" Hormone therapy might alleviate these problems, but the physician does not consider the issue important enough to even propose therapy.

One of the most important features of an active sex life in old age is having an interesting and interested partner. Researchers at Duke University in a longitudinal study of 254 men and women aged 60 to 94 found that 50 percent of the subjects in their sixties were still engaged in sexual activity and 10 to 20 percent of those in their eighties maintained sexual relations. The drop in activity in the seventies was due in part to physical illness, but the availability of partners becomes an issue at this age as well.[8] Women are particularly at a disadvantage because they usually outlive their husbands and have little chance of finding an available partner. Thus, in addition to the social and economic constraints faced by widows, they also lose the opportunity for sexual interaction. Nevertheless, in those fortunate individuals to whom an active sexual partner is still available there is no time limit drawn by the advancing years to their sexuality. Furthermore, the activity may be extending their lives.

4.
Heredity,
Parental Influences,
and Longevity

દ્⊸Genes influence the life span. This fact is suggested by comparisons of the life span between and within species. The life spans of each species of animal, including man, are fixed within the species, while varying dramatically between species. Since differences between species are genetically determined, the life span differences result primarily from genetic differences. From insects such as Ephermerids which live only a few hours, only long enough to reproduce, to man who can survive for over a century, to tortoises which can live for several hundred years, the maximum length of life is programmed by genetic factors. Individual differences in longevity existing within species have also been related to genetic differences. Long-lived and short-lived strains of animals have been bred; genealogies of long- and short-lived families have been traced; and individuals with the greatest genetic similarity—identical twins—have the most similar life spans.

As we explore some of the research which has indicated a relationship between heredity and longevity, it will become clear that the environment also plays a significant role in determining how the genetic influence is expressed. Thus, with humans, it is impossible to determine just how much of the parental influence on longevity is related to nutrition, education, health, and socioeconomic factors provided by parents, and how much parental influence results biologically from the genetic endowment which is also passed from parent to child. That genes affect longevity through secondary means, such as through intelligence, is also likely. Finally, physical factors such as parental age and birth order also show mild relationships with longevity.

Heredity and parental influence modify the length of our lives through a number of more or less direct pathways, but to understand how the mechanisms work we need more information than is available at present. Understanding of genetic mechanisms in longevity, which represents the aim of many biologists working in the field of aging, may enable us to alter the 120 year upper limit which appears to be set as man's genetic potential. While many gerontologists are not as optimistic as Dr. Bernard Strehler of the University of Southern Californa, who believes the genetic code for longevity may be broken within the next decade, many agree that the prospects for determining and altering the human life span are not longer in the realm of science fiction. In this chapter we will explore what is currently known about relationships between heredity, parental influence, and longevity, and in the Epilogue we will examine the prospects for further altering those relationships by modifying the genes.

LONGEVITY AND ANCESTRAL RELATIONSHIPS

Attempts to control environmental influences and to vary only genetic background have successfully demonstrated that within a given species there are genetic determinants of longevity. Naturally, this work has been undertaken only in subhuman species. Over twenty years ago, Dr. Alex Comfort reviewed the research on animal breeding for longevity and concluded that there is genetic control of the life span. While a number of species have been involved in such experiments, the breeding work becomes extremely difficult with anything longer-lived than a fruit fly because it is necessary to follow the offspring for several generations. Time and space do place natural limitations on such studies, but those carried out result in long-lived and short-lived strains. The only exception is that if inbreeding for longevity is carried on for many generations, the long-lived strains become shorter-lived from what is called "inbreeding depression." For the same reason that closely related humans (e.g., parents and children, brothers and sisters, first cousins) produce less vigorous, shorter-lived offspring, genetically similar animals which have been inbred for many generations produce less vigorous, shorter-lived offspring. Any recessive genes which are deleterious have a greater probability of being expressed when two closely related invididuals mate. Since in many parts of the world it is illegal for close relatives to marry and have children, the negative consequences of inbreeding for longevity are rarely expressed in humans.

Dr. Charles Goodrick of the Gerontology Research Center in Baltimore recently emphasized the importance of genetic influences in a study of the life spans and inheritance of longevity of inbred mice. He concluded that at least half of the variance associated with longevity is in all probability due to genetic factors. Environment undoubtedly plays a much greater role in human longevity than it does in the longevity of laboratory mice, but Goodrick's conclusions serve to emphasize the great significance of the role of genes in determining the life span.

Dr. Alex Comfort has reported a relationship between ancestral longevity and the longevity of offspring in studies of many species of animals *and* of humans. He maintains, however, that there is less correlation between human parents and their children for longevity than there is for height. In other words, although the children of long-lived parents are more likely to be long-lived, they are less likely to be so than the children of tall parents are likely to be tall. In the case of longevity, there are more exceptions to the rule than in the case of height—and we all know of cases of short children of tall parents and vice versa. Thus, if you have long-lived ancestors, your chances for long life are greater, but children of short-lived ancestors need not despair.

There are a number of problems with genealogical studies which make the results difficult to interpret. First, heredity is not the only factor involved. Families also provide more or less environmental supports which can affect longevity, and long life of a parent may produce a more favorable environment for offspring by allowing the parent to remain available for support. Conversely, loss of parents early in the lives of offspring might have negative consequences for longevity. In addition to the problem of interpreting how much of the ancestral contribution is genetic and how much is environmental, there are sampling problems with the genealogical studies. Information on the deaths of all family members is not always available, there are biases leading to the report of deaths primarily in young and middle adulthood, but not in childhood and old age, and all of the descendents sampled may not have died at the time the studies are undertaken.

Attempts were made by a number of researchers to control some of these factors. Those studied included a Massachusetts family, five centuries of a Chinese family, long-lived people in Baltimore, and Finnish nobility. All of these investigations had similar results. Children of long-lived parents and grandparents lived longer than children whose parents had died relatively young.

In one of these studies, Dr. Margaret Abbott of Johns Hopkins was careful not to rule out environmental explanations for these results, and in the process provided several possible interpretations of the fact that the longevity of the mother has a greater effect than that of the father on the offspring's longevity. One explanation is genetic. While the genetic material—the DNA—of the fertilized egg derives equally from both parents, the surrounding material in that cell, the cytoplasm, comes almost entirely from the mother. Thus, genetic factors in the cytoplasm might produce similarities between the mother and child which would not exist between the father and child. An environmental interpretation of these same results is that diet and cooking, patterns of exercise, attitudes toward life, and health habits are important to survival, and while both parents teach these practices and attitudes to their children, the mother may have more influence since she typically has closer contact with the children. Whether parents' and ancestors' influence on the longevity of offspring is genetic, environmental, or—more likely—an interaction of both, all the studies tend to provide convincing evidence of a genetic effect. Thus, we can predict to some degree our own life expectancy on the basis of how long our parents and grandparents have lived.

The most conclusive evidence that there is genetic component to longevity comes from studies comparing identical and fraternal twins. Identical twins develop from the same fertilized egg, thus their genetic make-up, the DNA in each cell of their bodies, is identical. Fraternal twins, however, have the same genetic relationship as siblings. Fraternal twinning is the result of two (instead of the usual one) ova being released during the same time-period, and each egg is fertilized by a different sperm. Franz Kallman and his associates have done extensive research with twins and longevity, and have found a greater concordance of longevity among identical than among fraternal twins. Since the environments for fraternal and identical twins are probably about equally similar, the primary difference between the two types of twins is genetic. The more genetically similar individuals die at more similar ages and of more similar causes. This point is made dramatically in some of the case histories reported by Dr. Kallman and his associate, Dr. G. Sander. In one case, identical twin sisters with very different life patterns died within a month of one another of the same cause. One of the sisters remained single throughout her entire life, while the other married and became the mother of a large number of children. Both died at the age of sixty-nine within a month of one another after both had a cerebral hemorrhage at the same time. Another case is reported of identical twin brothers who died at the age of eighty-six on the same day. While these two cases are remarkable for the extremely close time interval within which the two members of the identical twin pair died, many other cases of identical twins have been reported in which both members died within a one to three year period. The point is that identical twins who have identical genetic make-up resemble one another remarkably throughout life in their physical appearances, behavior, and longevity, and such resemblance provides strong evidence for genetic contribution to all of those features.

Is there a gene which codes for longevity, or is longevity determined by multiple genes? Because the hereditary patterns for longevity do not conform to those which would be prevalent if a single gene were operating, it appears that multiple genes are involved. However, Dr. R. G. Cutler has suggested that the number of genes coding for life span in humans may not be large. He feels that only a few genes are responsible for the age changes observed in many different physiological functions, suggesting that only a few of the hundreds of thousands of genes parents pass on to children are coded for longevity. Such a conclusion also suggests that the task of altering the genetic code for longevity may not be as great as had been anticipated.

PARENTAL AGE AND BIRTH ORDER

In addition to the cultural and genetic heritage we receive from our parents, we are also affected by our parents' ages at the time of our birth. Children born of relatively young parents survive longer than children born late in the lives of the parents. The effect appears to be related more to the mother's than to the father's age at birth of the child, but since individuals usually marry people around their same age, it is difficult to separate maternal and paternal effects in humans. In animal studies, the older the mother, the shorter-lived were the offspring. It has long been known that neonatal mortality, premature births, and stillbirths are more frequent in mothers over the age of 35. Likewise, the children of older mothers who do survive at birth still have shorter life expectancies than children of younger mothers. The offspring of older mothers are at much greater risk for Mongolism and malformations of various kinds, in addition to the other risks mentioned above. It has also been demonstrated that *very* young mothers (under 18) have more abnormal births and presumably shorter-lived children.

The explanations proffered for the negative effects of births very early and very late in the mother's life have been both biological and social-psychological, and no one explanation has generally been accepted. From a biological point of view, it may be that the reproductive apparatus of very young and very old mothers is not in the same prime condition as the reproductive system of 18-35 year old mothers. Social-psychological explanations of the fact that children of very young and old mothers have shorter life expectancies involve the notion that mothers in these ages are less suited for motherhoood, and as a result may not provide the best care for their children. This hypothesis is difficult to defend in the case of older women, who may be in an ideal position to provide the emotional support and patient, loving care required to maximize develooment in offspring. The social-psychological approach is also inadequate in explaining the greater neonatal mortality rates for both younger and older mothers.

Before we leave the topic of maternal age and longevity, one more fact should be considered. Over the last century the number of years in which a woman can conceive and bear children has been progressively extended. Menopause is coming later in the life span of women, and as more of us mainatin our health into later years, while postponing marriage and chidlbearing later and later, it may become more common for first children to be born to women in their 30's and even 40's. Would this situation then shorten the life expectancy of future generations? Perhaps. However, it might also be the case that improvments in health care and nutrition make us more fit to bear children later. Furthermore, the data we now have on women who bear children late in life may be negatively biased, representing women who had problems conceiving and bearing children during the "prime" years and who only became pregnant after many miscarriages or abortions. As it becomes more of a cultural norm to postpone childbearing, with the healthiest and most successful women waiting later to conceive, a different pattern of infant mortality in older mothers may appear. Besides, with techniques such as amniocentesis (a safe medical procedure which permits the obstetrician to examine the chromosomes of the fetus) it is now possible to detect genetic aberrations such as Mongolism before the baby is born. In the case of Mongolism and other serious genetic defects the mother can abort the young fetus and avoid bearing an abnormal baby. In the future, it may be possible to detect faulty fetuses and repair the damage with genetic engineering before birth. Even in the present, however, modern techniques have dramatically reduced the risks of childbearing for older mothers, and older mothers themselves may be in less danger than they have been in previous decades.

As noted previously, it is generally agreed that maternal age has a greater effect on a child's life expectancy than does paternal age. What is not clear is if paternal age has an effect at all. There have been a number of studies on the subject, none of them conclusive. There is some indication that the effect of paternal age on longevity may be slightly negative, but if there is any effect at all, it is so small that it is frequently not apparent.

In addition to the observed relationship between the age of parents and longevity, it has been noted that birth order is related to long life, a result which has been replicated a number of times. The results show that the earlier in the birth order a child is born, the longer he or she is likely to live. It is difficult to determine if this finding results solely from the parental age effect (the older the parents, the less likely the child is to be first-born), or if it is a separate effect. Birth order may be the maternal age effect in another form, or it may be that even if maternal age is controlled the mother's reproductive capacity with later children may be poorer than with the first and second. Another explanation might be that the first born have more cultural advantages. They receive more attention and esteem from the parents and are thus better prepared and better protected. Whatever the explanation, the effect does occur, and it is another means by which we can predict an individual's life expectancy.

INTELLIGENCE, GENES, AND LONGEVITY

While the relative contribution of genes to intellectual ability is a very controversial topic, few scientists argue that intellectual endowment has no genetic component. The data on the inheritability of IQ are just too convincing. The correlation between the IQ scores of unrelated individuals is zero, and with increasing degree of genetic similarity, the correlations between IQ scores of individuals increase. Thus, the IQ scores of biological parents and children are much more alike than the IQ scores of foster parents and children, even when the child has never seen its biological parents. The IQ scores of full siblings are more similar than half siblings, and the IQ scores of fraternal twins, having the same magnitude of genetic similarity as siblings are about as similar as the IQ scores of siblings. The most convincing evidence for genetic contribution to IQ scores comes from studies of identical twins reared both together and apart. There is an extremely high concordance between the IQ scores of identical twins, even when reared apart. This concordance of identical twins' IQ scores continues at all ages throughout the life span, including toward the end of life, when an individual's IQ scores drops precipitously around two years before death—the IQ scores of identical twins tend to show the drop around the same time.

We have already discussed the fact that there is a genetic component to longevity, and now evidence has been presented that there is a genetic component to intelligence. It is also true that people of high intelligence live longer. Thus, having genes which code for long life may also predispose the individual to be more intelligent—or perhaps having a high intelligence leads a person to adopt strategies and attain status favorable to long life.

It is true that people who have experienced social and economic advantages will score higher on intelligence tests, and this is part of the reason that higher intelligence is related to longer life. People of low socioeconomic status have neither the opportunity nor the access to experiences and resources which lead individuals to score higher on intelligence tests. However, the correlation between longevity and intelligence appears to be more than simply an environmental opportunity effect. Among bright people in general the very brightest live longest. This is the reason we have stipulated that your IQ must be *very* high in order to add an extra 2 years to your life. People with above average intelligence are already going to receive extra years on the test in categories such as education, occupation, and income. In order to receive an advantage beyond that there must be a genetic advantage operating in which the person is really unusually gifted with regard to intelligence.

The evidence for this extra advantage for very bright people comes from several different types of studies. The Metropolitan Life Insurance Company undertook the first study showing this effect in 1932. Assessing longevity in male college graduates from eight Eastern colleges, it was found that college graduates had a higher life expectancy than the general white male population. Even more significant, honor students—those students who had done the most outstanding work among the college graduates—had an even better life expectancy. Assuming that the honor graduates were in the exceptionally intelligent category, this suggests that exceptional intelligence adds years to the life span.

A long-term study of exceptionally bright individuals provides additional evidence that very high intelligence plays a role in longevity. In California in the 1930's, Dr. Louis Terman undertook a longitudinal study of the very brightest school-children in the state. He selected only children who scored above 140 on the Stanford-Binet intelligence test (considered a superior range of intelligence). There were over a thousand children included in the study, and Terman and his associates followed these individuals as they grew into adolescence and adulthood. These gifted individuals are currently in their 60's and 70's, and the information collected on them over their lives has been published in five volumes (called *Genetic Studies of Genius*). The results show that the group is superior in many ways (less mental illness, fewer divorces, brighter children, greater occupational success), including longevity. They are dying in much smaller numbers than would be predicted from the general population. Thus, again, very high intelligence appears to contribute to longer life.

Many people dislike the idea that phenomena such as longevity and intelligence are affected by heredity. They feel that if the effect is genetic, then it is immutable. However, this is not the case. While we are not yet at a stage in science where we can actually alter the genes, we can intervene at other levels and alter the effect of the genes. This is clearly shown in the case of diabetes mellitus which is inherited: although we cannot prevent a child from having the disease, we can treat the child with insulin so that he or she leads a nearly normal life. In the case of heart disease, which is also known to run in families, we can alter the diet and lifestyle of individuals to help them avoid the risk. In the case of intelligence, the genes set a range or potential which environmental advantages can maximize. In the next chapter, we will examine how to maximize our chances for long life, regardless of our heritage.

5.
What You Can Do About The Effects of Heredity on Longevity: Preventive Medicine

᪣One of the natural assumptions people make when considering how heredity affects their life expectancy is that the influence is irreversible and inevitable. Since we cannot choose our parents or grandparents, and hence our genes, we are likely to assume that hereditary weaknesses predisposing us to cancer, strokes, or heart attacks have to be accepted as part of our fate. Such an assumption is a mistake. Indeed, it can be a fatal mistake.

In the last twenty years a great deal has been learned about the risk factors involved in the major killing diseases in the United States: coronary heart disease and cancer. Many of the habits and lifestyle patterns of Americans appear to contribute to these diseases, and changing these patterns can increase life expectancy. Thus, while parents and grandparents who died of these diseases at an early age may have had a genetic weakness for them, they may also have unknowingly contributed to their early demise through their lifestyle. By educating ourselves with the knowledge we now have about risk factors, we can avoid these dangerous patterns. In this manner we are in a position to neutralize the effect of the genetic predisposition and beat the odds handed down in our genes.

Those of us who are smug about the fact that our ancestors survived to a ripe old age should not skip the rest of this chapter. Heredity is only one of the many factors which determines the development of coronary heart disease. As pictured schematically in Figure 4, coronary heart disease results as the end stage of a life-long process. The first stage, in which the individual develops chronically high levels of cholesterol in the blood, results as an interaction between diet and heredity aggravated by obesity. That many Americans have such a genetic predisposition for hypercholesterolemia (high blood serum cholesterol level) is evidenced by the fact that half of the deaths in the United States result from coronary heart disease. A number of studies tracing family-related patterns of heart disease have also documented the genetic component, and it is rather prevalent in our population. With time, after hypercholesterolemia has developed, and in coexistence with other risk factors such as hypertension (high blood pressure), atherosclerosis (a build-up of fatty substances in the arteries) occurs—without any noticeable symptoms. Cigarette smoking, stress, and physical inactivity added to (and probably worsening) this atherosclerosis result in clinically detectable coronary heart disease.

Lifestyle and health habits play a significant role regardless of our genetic background, and many of the leading causes of death in later life present some potential for control and prevention. Diseases of the cardiovascular system and cancer account for about 70 percent of the deaths in the United States each year, and the majority of these deaths do not result only from a genetic predisposition for the diseases. All of us are at risk for some form of heart disease and cancer, but we could greatly reduce our risk if we adopted certain health habits, food preferences, and life patterns early in our lives and taught them to our children from birth.

FIGURE 4. The Conceptualized Stages and Critical Factors in the Development of Coronary Heart Disease.

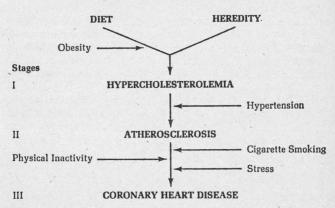

SOURCE: W. F. Connor, and S. L. Connor, "The Key Role of Nutritional Factors in the Prevention of Coronary Heart Disease," *Preventive Medicine*, 1972, 1, 49–83.

PREVENTIVE ACTION IN CORONARY HEART DISEASE

As stated previously, the number one cause of death in the United States is disease involving the heart and blood vessels. This includes heart attacks, strokes, and various diseases of the cardiovascular system. It has been estimates that one to three million Americans had heart disease in 1975, and 675,000 of these people with identifiable heart problems will die from them in the next several years. On the positive side, cardiovascular disease is primarily a disease of middle and old age and has become the major cause of death because we have been able to control infectious diseases which used to kill more of us before we reached middle age. On the negative side, cardiovascular disease appears to be the product of industrialization and modern society.

At least one authority, Dr. T. M. Peery, believes that coronary heart disease should be looked at as a new disease, and that we should seek its cause among conditions that developed during the 1920's and 1930's. This is due to the fact that before 1930 heart attack was rarely diagnosed; today it is the leading cause of death. To account for the remarkable rise in heart attacks, Peery considers three factors: smoking, greater consumption of meat and dairy products, and lack of exercise. He concurs with most experts that changes in diet and exercise are the major causal factors. Stress, inactivity, and caloric excess all contribute heavily to the onset of heart disease. These factors, like medical advances, seem to accompany "advances" in civilization. Fortunately, all of these negative factors can come under our control.

Risk Factors in Heart Disease

Two specialists in heart disease and preventive medicine, Dr. Jeremiah Stamler and Dr. Frederick Epstein, recently stated that candidates for the future development of premature coronary heart disease can now be identified with a certainty unsurpassed for most other diseases. They feel that the predictability of heart disease in middle age from simple risk factor measurements provides an enormous potential for curbing this contemporary epidemic. Furthermore, they assert that the eventual elimination of this disease demands, in addition to identification and care of the susceptible individuals, changes in the mode of life of most people in the United States. Given that our very lives are at stake, it is surprising that Americans are so unwilling to make the necessary changes. Let us examine what they entail.

The three best predictors of heart disease, or the major risk factors, are: (1) high blood cholesterol level, (2) high blood pressure, and (3) cigarette smoking. Other risk factors which may be casually related to these three major predictors of heart attack are diet, lack of exercise, and a hard-driving, aggressive personality. Diabetes also makes an individual more prone to heart attacks. Each factor alone increases the risk to the individual of having a heart attack in mid-life, and when two or more of the factors are present together in one person the risk increases vastly.

The first risk factor, blood serum cholesterol level, can be determined through a laboratory test obtained at your doctor's office. It was stressed in the life expectancy test that it is important to get a physical examination annually, and one of the things which can be determined at this examination is if you are at risk for cardiovascular disease. A simple test to determine if you have a high level of cholesterol in your blood will alert you as to whether you need to modify your diet.

What serum cholesterol level is safe? The data indicate that there is a steady increment in the risk of a heart attack as the cholesterol level rises. Thus, the answer is, the lower the level, the lower the risk. There seems to be no clear cut-off point. The clinical practice is to use a level of less than 200 mg/dl as normal, 200-249 mg/dl as borderline risk, and 250 mg/dl or above as high risk. Clearly, this should not make the individual with a serum cholesterol level of 248 mg/dl breathe a sigh of relief. This person is at greater risk than someone at 210 mg/dl, who in turn as a greater chance of having a heart attack than a person with a serum cholesterol level of 160 mg/dl.

Because it is still unclear as to exactly how cholesterol level is involved in cardiovascular disease, there has been some controversy as to whether we should all be trying to reduce the cholesterol in our diet. Other internal factors have been suggested by some as better predictors of heart disease. While there is no definitive answer as of the present time, it appears that cholesterol is at least as good a predictor as the other measures, so the safest practice is to keep our blood cholesterol levels down, and the proper diet helps to do this.

High blood pressure is another factor which places an individual at serious risk for a heart attack. Like serum cholesterol level, the higher the blood pressure, the greater the risk. Blood pressure is another measure which is usually assessed in a medical facility, and it is important to be aware of your own blood pressure level and any changes occurring in it over the year.

Blood pressure is measured in two parts. Systolic pressure, the higher number, is the pressure in the arteries at the peak of a heart beat, when the heart is pumping the blood out. Diastolic pressure is the pressure at the low point of the heart cycle, at the interval between the strokes. Diastolic and systolic blood pressure measurements are highly correlated, and similar predictions for heart attacks are made with each measure. Drs. Stamler and Epstein reported predictions on the basis of diastolic pressure, and since this measure may be a little more stable than systolic pressure, it is more frequently chosen. People with a diastolic blood pressure of 105 mm/Hg are four times as likely to have a heart attack as those with a diastolic pressure below 75 mm/Hg. Maintaining diastolic blood pressure below 85 mm/Hg appears to have a positive effect on longevity, and even modest elevations in diastolic blood pressure (85-94 mm/Hg) are associated with gross increases in risk. Thus, maintaining diastolic blood pressure below 85 mm/Hg appears to be relatively safe, with a pressure below 75 mm/Hg being even less of a risk. The diastolic blood pressure which is optimal for longevity is 70 mm/Hg, and low-risk systolic pressure is 120 mm/Hg or below.

We all know the association between smoking and lung cancer, but fewer of us are aware that smoking is one of the major risk factors in heart disease as well. For those who regularly smoke cigarettes, the risk rises steadily with the number of cigarettes smoked per day. The relationship is quantitative and continuous. There is twice as much risk for those who smoke more than a pack a day than for those smoking a pack a day or less. Such a direct relationship clearly implies that cigarette smoking is causing heart attacks. People who have quit smoking have a slightly greater risk than those who have never smoked, but those who smoke more than a pack a day have almost three times the risk for a heart attack as those who have quit smoking. There is no question that smokers can do something which dramatically reduces their risk of a heart attack. QUIT.

Unfortunately, the average American has at least one of these three major risk factors. In Stamler and Epstein's study of 7,342 American males, 83 percent were high on at least one of the risk factors. Since having one risk factor made an individual over twice as prone to a heart attack as those who had no risk factors, a great majority of these men were at least twice as vulnerable to heart attack as the men who practiced better health and dietary habits. Having two of the three risk factors was even more dangerous, causing four times the risk for heart attack—almost a third of the men in Stamler and Epstein's sample had two of the risk factors.

Eight percent of the sample had all three of the risk factors, making them more than eight times as likely to have a heart attack and more than five times as likely to die of it. Detection of these factors and alleviation of the risk could extend the life expectancy dramatically.

What are your chances as an individual to develop coronary heart disease? Dr. H. M. Whyte has recently calculated the risk for individuals on the basis of data collected on a population living in Framingham, Mass., who have been observed over a considerable portion of their adult life span. The risks are broken down by cholesterol level, age, sex, and association with other measured risk factors, including cigarette smoking and high blood pressure. (Statistics reported were computed assuming that glucose tolerance level is normal, and that there is no identifiable damage in the heart.) After your annual physical check-up, ask your physician for your systolic blood pressure and cholesterol levels. With this information you can predict your own chances for heart attack and you can also undertake preventive measures to put yourself in a lower category of risk. Individualized risk factors are presented in Table 1. Find your risk by looking up the correct row for your sex, age, and cholesterol level under the column matching your smoking habits and systolic blood pressure (high blood pressure here is measured at 165 mm/Hg and above). For example, if you are a 45-year-old woman with a cholesterol level of 200 who does not smoke, and who has a systolic blood pressure of 120 (which is below the high-risk level for blood pressure), you have a 5 percent chance of developing coronary heart disease in the next twenty years.

Well-tested means of correcting the three major risk factors are available—diet for high cholesterol level, diet (weight control and moderate salt restriction) and drugs (when necessary) for high blood pressure, and elimination of smoking. Stamler and Epstein estimated that if all of the men with two or three risk factors would have agreed to eliminate one or two or three risk factors, the mortality rate in that sample would have been cut in half. If such a reduction in mortality rate is projected for all young and middle-aged men in the United States—who die at a rate of 150,000 a year from coronary deaths—40,000 lives per year would be saved. If all of us changed our habits so as to eliminate all risk factors the

TABLE 1.

Smoking		Cholesterol	No	No	Yes	Yes
High blood pressure			No	Yes	No	Yes
Sex	Age	Cholesterol mg/100 ml	Percent of individuals developing coronary heart disease in 20 years			
Male	35	310	13.5	22.0	20.8	32.6
		260	8.4	14.1	13.3	21.6
		210	5.1	8.9	8.4	13.9
	45	310	22.5	35.2	33.5	49.5
		260	16.9	27.0	25.7	39.4
		210	12.6	20.6	19.6	30.7
	55	310	23.9	37.0	35.2	51.5
		260	20.9	32.7	31.1	46.4
		210	18.2	28.9	27.6	41.8
Female	45	310	9.1	16.4	9.6	17.2
		260	6.7	12.4	7.2	13.1
		210	5.1	9.6	5.5	10.1
	55	310	14.9	26.1	15.7	27.4
		260	11.8	21.2	12.5	22.2
		210	9.4	17.0	9.9	18.0

SOURCE: Modified from Whyte, 1975 (Whyte, H. M., "Potential Effect on Coronary-Heart-Disease Morbidity of Lowering the Blood-Cholesterol," *Lancet*, 1975, 1, 906–910.

savings in lives would be enormous, and the average life expectancy would increase dramatically. Chances are many more of us would live to be 100.

In addition to the major risk factors, there are other factors associated with a higher risk for cardiovascular disease which act somewhat independently of the three major factors. Eating the typical rich American diet often leads to obesity, which in itself may stress the heart and blood vessels. Our sedentary lifestyle also contributes to obesity, and even in slim individuals it has been found that moderate exercise which enhances fitness in the heart and lungs is associated with fewer heart attacks. Personality and behavior patterns have also been associated with cardiovascular disease. It appers that the American ideal, the upwardly mobile, hard-driving individual who is constantly on the go, is just the type most likely to have a heart attack. In our society we almost seem to condition people to stress their cardiovascular systems. Each of these risk factors, obesity, exercise, and personality, along with the means for their control is treated individually in following chapters.

How to Eliminate the Major Risk Factors in Heart Disease

There is no mystery involved in how to eliminate one of the biggest risk factors in heart disease (and also a risk factor in cancer), smoking. There is clear evidence that quitting smoking helps to alleviate the risk. However, if you cannot quit, then at least cut down on the number of cigarettes smoked. Since there is a direct relationship between the number of cigarettes smoked and the incidence of heart disease, the more you can cut down the better. Any effort you make to cut back your smoking will help.

One of the alarming trends in the United States is the increase in smoking among adolescents and young adults. While the Public Health Service warnings about the dangers of cigarette smoking appear to have reached many in adulthood, younger people in great numbers are still being seduced into the habit of smoking. Perhaps their feeling is that they have so much of their lives left to life that the years which will be cut off by cigarette smoking do not matter. Such attitudes must be changed. Both the quality and quantity of life are affected by cigarette smoking.

Many means of cutting or ending cigarette consumption exist. Products such as a series of increasingly strong filters are sold in the drug store and supermarket. Clinics to aid in terminating smoking habits abound. Many individuals decide to quit and carry it out on their own with only the aid of their willpower and the tremendous gratitude of those whom they subjected to this polluting habit. For a woman, quitting the smoking habit is the single greatest thing she can do to extend her life expectancy. Apart from castration—which is not a viable solution— there is nothing a man can do which will extend his life expectancy more than to quit smoking.

Alleviating the risk factors of high cholesterol level and

high blood pressure require several steps which include consultation with a physician. The first step is to have a physical examination to determine what these levels are. Then, with the guidance of your physician, you can work to keep the levels under control.

High cholesterol level is affected by diet, and fortunately it can nearly always be alleviated by a change in diet. Basically, to lower cholesterol level a calorie-controlled diet is necessary, one which is low in saturated fat and cholesterol, moderate in total fat and carbohydrate, and moderate in polyunsaturated fat. Most physicians will prescribe a diet for you to reduce cholesterol, and you can also find low-cholesterol diets in many books on health and diet. (See Appendix for chart showing cholesterol content for selected foods.)

Because high cholesterol level is induced by the usual U.S. diet does not mean that there is no genetic factor involved. In many Americans who have problems with high cholesterol level, the disease is due to genetic metabolic abnormalities. This fact should sensitize those who are aware that their parents have high cholesterol levels and those parents who know that their cholesterol level is high to protect their families from this disease. Children inherit both their parents' genes and their living habits. Living habits can be changed, and changing a habit such as diet clearly neutralizes the genetic predisposition to high cholesterol level. Thus, to practice preventative medicine to its fullest, individuals who have been identified as having high cholesterol levels should alert family members and change the eating patterns of the whole family.

High blood pressure can be controlled through diet and drugs, and moderate exercise (which helps us to relax) has also been shown to lower blood pressure. It is essential to work with your physician in the case of high blood pressure. You may need to go on a diet to reduce your weight, and your physician should prescribe the kind of weight-loss diet which is best suited to your needs. The physician may also suggest that you lower your salt intake. If your blood pressure is more than moderately high, your physician may prescribe medication. Drugs can safely reduce the level of blood pressure, and many individuals benefit for years by taking medication for this problem. The important first step, however, is to identify the problem. Many Americans have high blood pressure and are unaware of it. This seems to be especially true of blacks. Men are more at risk for hypertension up to the age of 50; after that age, women are more likely to be hypertensive than men. This may be related to hormonal changes which occur in women after menopause.

Exceedingly simple measures are needed to determine blood pressure, and relatively simple and safe procedures are available to control hypertension. Thus, it is senseless for so many of us to continue to live with this risk factor which has been compared to a time bomb. High pressure in the arteries can in a sense lead to an explosion, resulting in a stroke or heart attack, leaving an individual permanently paralyzed, grossly restricted in terms of activity, or dead.

In the face of this extremely clear evidence, why are so many of us reluctant to take the precautions necessary to extend our lives? Why is it so difficult even so much as to get ourselves to a physician once a year—let alone change our eating habits or quit smoking? The answer seems to be that most of us believe that statistics are computed on the basis of other people's lives—not our own. We see ourselves as different, less vulnerable. *We* never participated in a study on heart disease, so *we* are not included in those statistics. This is such a false illusion. Clearly 83 percent of the very large sample of men in Drs. Stamler and Epstein's study had at least one risk factor. Do we seriously believe that we all really belong to the 17 percent who are not high in any of the risk categories? The smokers among us *know* they are at risk, and few of the rest of us would take 8-to-2 odds on any bet. It's really time to stop kidding ourselves and to let ourselves be counted among those who are at risk. Just acknowledging the risk is the hardest part. Once this step is taken, we can control the risk and count ourselves among those who have the best chance of living to be 100.

Very dramatic evidence that heart disease can be reduced by the measures described above was reported in *The New York Times* (April 3, 1977). A rural county in eastern Finland, North Karelia, had the highest heart disease rate in the world. Concerned community leaders petitioned the national government for help, and in 1972 the Finnish government, with the help of the World Health Organization, supported a program involving the entire North Karelia population of 180,000. After five years the program has been a tremendous success—the heart attack rate for males has dropped 40 percent, and the trend over the past 30 years for an annual increase in heart attacks has been reversed. North Karelia has dropped to fifth in terms of heart attack rate among the counties of Finland.

The change in the rate of heart attack was achieved with a massive program directed at the three major predictors of heart attack: high blood cholesterol, high blood pressure, and smoking. A team of 15—half medical and the rest economists, sociologists, psychologists, and individuals working in related professions—headed by Dr. Pekka Puska evaluated the results and involved the entire community in various projects.

Laws were passed forbidding smoking in public buildings and on public transportation, and many private businesses enforced similar laws in their offices. Newspapers and radio stations, leaflets and posters, all publicized the risk for heart attack involved with smoking. Such efforts led to a 10 percent reduction in the number of men who smoked.

Changing the diet was more difficult as the North Karelian diet is traditionally based on fatty foods. The dairy was the first line of attack as Dr. Puska felt that dairy products were a key source of fat. An attempt was made to get residents to switch from whole milk to low-fat milk and finally to skim milk. The dairy cooperated by promoting low fat and skim milk. Bread thickly spread with butter was another traditional North Karelian staple. The people were encouraged to use margarine. They were also asked to give up the popular grilled sausages which contained a great deal of fat. A substitute for the local product was developed using mushrooms which grow plentifully in the surrounding forests. The sausages now contain 25 percent mushroom content, and they sell very well. Fresh vegetables were a rarity in the diet of the North Karelians, so they were encouraged to add vegetables to their diet. At least some of these measures were successful. Users of low-fat milk increased from 17 to 56 percent and users of butter decreased from 86 to 69 percent.

The most difficult risk factor to control was high blood pressure. Attempts were made to detect high blood pressure early in the lives of these Finnish people, and everyone in the community was screened for blood pressure at frequent intervals. In a number of cases, drug treatment was administered to lower blood pressure.

By undertaking this major effort, a number of lives in the community were saved. Indeed, the heart attack rate in the community was almost cut in half. Such a program attests to the fact that preventative measures work and can be carried out on a large scale. While we are not yet ready in the United States to invest in such a massive public program of preventative medicine, as individuals we can carry out the same changes in our lives as practiced by the Finns. And like them, we will live longer.

PREVENTIVE ACTION IN CANCER

Like heart disease, certain forms of cancer appear to run in families. However, cancer is much more than just a hereditary disease. It is the second greatest killer in the United States; one out of four people now living will develop some kind of cancer, and of these individuals two-thirds will die within five years of the diagnosis. It has been estimated that half of all persons with cancer could be cured by earlier diagnosis and full use of medical facilities, because we know many of the causes of cancer, and in a number of additional cases we can control the disease once it is detected. Thus, like cardiovascular disease, cancer is a disease which with preventive measures, can be controlled far better than it is currently.

Risk Factors in Cancer and Their Elimination

The general characteristic of cancer is a proliferation of foreign cells in the body which interfere with the function of normal cells. There are a number of different kinds of cancers, and they appear to be associated with different risk factors. Cancer appears to progress in three stages: at first the cancer is small and localized to a small area of the body; the second state occurs when it expands to cover a whole region of the body; and final stage is when it had advanced throughout the body, and at this stage of widespread cancer death is almost inevitable.

Since the characteristic common to all cancers is the tendency to expand, to proliferate and extend to large areas of the body, the most general preventative measure in the case of cancer is early detection. Cancer must be found early in its onset if lives are to be saved. An annual physical examination is as important in the detection of cancer as it is in the detection of risk factors in heart disease. In men, cancer of the prostate, colon, and rectum are among the top seven causes of cancer deaths, and detection of these cancers is made with proctoscopic examination. Such an examination should be made at least every two years in adult males and it should be made annually for men over the age of 40. Breast cancer is the leading cause of cancer death among women, and it can be detected early and successfully treated. Women should learn to give themselves a monthly breast self-examination and have an annual physical exam. A Pap test for uterine cancer and a pelvic examination for ovarian cancer should also be carried out, since mortality from cancer in the genital areas and in the urinary tract is high for both men and women, and can be detected and controlled with annual examinations.

Lung cancer, the leading cause of cancer death in men, has been positively linked to cigarette smoking. Unfortunately, fewer then one in every ten persons in whom lung cancer is diagnosed is saved. However, three out of four cases of lung cancer could be prevented in the first place if men and women would stop smoking, thus eliminating the major cause of lung cancer and preventing countless unnecessary deaths.

Another risk which has been associated with lung cancer is air pollution. Comparing individuals living in rural and urban areas it has been found that the lung cancer rate in non-polluted areas is much lower. In an article on air pollution and human health, Dr. Lester Lave and Dr. Eugene Seskin estimated that 25 percent of the deaths from lung cancer could be eliminated by reducing air pullution by 50 percent. Air pollution has also been associated with mortality from forms of cancer other than lung cancer. Thus, while we cannot as individuals do much about air pollution, we can make a decision to escape it and move to areas which are not so polluted.

Those exposed to pollutants through their occupation are particularly at risk with regard to lung cancer and cancer in general. Especially vulnerable are asbestos workers, printers, typographers, cotton mill workers, vinyl chloride workers, and roofers. Even those living near asbestos manufacturing plants have a greater cancer risk. Industries with such risk rates must be forced to take adequate steps to protect their workers, and individuals interested in living to a ripe old age are best advised to avoid these risky occupations.

Sun worshipers should be aware of the danger of cancer of the skin. While relatively few cancer deaths occur as a result of skin cancer, it is a problem which can be avoided by simply limiting the amount of explosure to the sun.

Cancer of the stomach, a major cause of cancer death, appears to be on the decline over the last decade. Some studies have linked stomach cancer to diet. A diet high in starchy foods and low in fresh vegetables and fruits appears to be associated with stomach cancer. Drs. M. Hakama and E. A. Saxen found an association with cereal consumption and stomach cancer. In countries where more cereal and flour is used, the incidence of stomach cancer is greater.

The other type of food which has been most associated with cancer incidence is fat consumption and meat and animal protein consumption which are highly related to fat consumption. Cancer of the colon, rectum, bladder, pancreas, breast, uterus, ovaries, prostate, and testes has been associated with high fat or animal protein consumption.

Cancer is a disease which has increased in incidence in modern society, partly because it is a disease of middle and late life and is experienced by more of us because we are surviving in greater numbers to middle and older age. Some of the vices of modern society such as air pollution and smoking also account for its greater prevalence in modern times. Indeed, many researchers feel that environmental factors such as asbestos dust, cigarette smoke, pollutants, viruses, radiation, and food additives account for 80 percent of cancers.

There is some question as to whether the incidence of cancer is rising. In 1975 the national statistics indicated an increase of 3 percent in cancer mortality, while data for Metropolitan Standard Ordinary life insurance policyholders, which are adjusted for changes in the age and sex distribution of the population from one year to the next, showed a 2 percent reduction in cancer mortality for 1975. With basic research on cancer making some strides in determining how the disease is triggered, and with medical advances in surgical, irradiation, and chemical treatment techniques, it appears that we are on the way to conquering cancer. With all these advances, however, it is still essential to detect the disease in an early state in order to successfully treat it. Thus, in addition to abandoning cigarette smoking, the single biggest step we can take in preventing cancer from shortening our lives is to have an annual medical examination.

HEALTH

6.
Body Weight and Diet for Long Life

There is little question that obesity shortens life expectancy. There is also general agreement that nutrition influences health and longevity. The maintenance of a moderate caloric intake with the proper balance of nutrients is a common feature in the lifestyle of extremely long-lived people in such diverse regions as Ecuador, Pakistan, and Russia. Alexander Leaf who has spent much of his scientific career studying these peoples feels that diet may be one of the important keys to their longevity. In animal research one of the very few manipulations which has worked to extend the life span, the upper limit of years for the species, involves diet. Animals fed a restricted number of calories early in life will exceed the life span for their species. While underfeeding probably does not have the same dramatic effect in humans, there are nutritional interventions which work to help people to come closer to their genetic potential for longevity. At the very least, the information presently available on nutrition, obesity, and longevity can help us to stop killing ourselves at an early age.

OBESITY—A MULTIFACETED KILLER

The average American is overweight. In our society of overabundance, we are actually committing suicide by trying to eat up our surplus. Over-consumption is costing us years of our lives. It has been estimated that if overweight and its related diseases were eliminated in the United States, four years would be added to the average life expectancy. This may even be an underestimate of the benefit of eliminating obesity, since many conditions known to decrease life expectancy are less severe when uncomplicated by excess weight.

It is a matter of accepted fact in our society that we increase in weight as we move from adolescence to young adulthood to middle age. Many weight charts based on average American weights indicate that normal weight can increase with age. Since these charts are based on "average" data, and since "average" Americans are overweight to begin with, maintaining our weight within the limits of these charts gives us a false sense of security. As we age the percent of our bodies which is muscle decreases, and the percent comprised of fat increases. Thus, to maintain the same muscle-fat ratio throughout our lives, we should actually lose weight as we grow older.

Consider the weight you were around the age of eighteen. If you were not overweight at that point in your life (and fewer of us were), for you to be in optimal health today your weight should be the same or a few pounds lighter than your weight as an eighteen-year-old. Returning to this weight will help you to avoid the very large number of risks you run as an overweight or obese person.

Tragically, many parents foster obesity in their children from infancy. A plump baby is considered a healthy one, and parents who have fat babies are praised for their excellent care. Such parents who promote overweight in infants and children are setting the stage for a lifetime of problems—psychological, social, and physical. We are born with a fixed number of cells which store body fat, but it is possible to increase this number of fat cells by overeating. And once we increase the number of fat cells, we cannot eliminate them. They will be with us the rest of our lives, and their existence will trigger mechanisms causing our appetite to increase, thus setting up a vicious cycle.

The effect of childhood obesity on weight in later life has been studied in Hagerstown, Maryland, in a population which has been followed by the Public Health Service since the 1920's. In 1971 a report was issued on the results of a follow-up study of 717 white males who had first been examined between 1923 and 1928 when they were from 9 to 13 years old. They were in their 40's at the time of the follow-up study. There was a striking tendency for overweight children to be overweight adults. No less that 84 percent of the men who had been overweight in childhood were still overweight as middle-aged adults. The study also showed the tendency of Americans to become overweight as they age. Fifty percent of the below average weight children became average or overweight adults. Forty percent of the men who were of average weight as children were overweight as adults, and 60 percent who had been moderately overweight as children were overweight adults. Thus, parents who overfeed their children make it almost impossible for the children to be slim as adults. Indeed, even many of the thin children became overweight adults, a pattern which had deleterious effects on health. The individuals in the Hagerstown study who were the most prone to hypertension were the men who had been below or average weight as children and had become overweight as adults. This pattern of becoming overweight in middle age is now the norm in the United States. As has been noted, such a pattern is most likely to lead us to high blood pressure, which is a major risk factor for heart attack and other diseases of the heart and vascular system.

Over 25 years ago Dr. Clive McCay, working at Cornell University, reported some of the first experimental evidence of the deleterious effects of obesity. Overfeeding rats and causing them to become obese led them to suffer an increased incidence of all kinds of age-associated diseases, including diseases of the lungs and kidney, and tumors. While many of the diseases which kill humans are different from the diseases which kill rats, the effect of obesity in humans is generally the same as it is in rats. It clearly increases the incidence of disease. Many diseases which are the killers in old age are directly caused or secondarily complicated by obesity. The overweight individual is more prone to suffer from a number of ailments, among them; bronchitis, diabetes, gallstones, gout, hypertension, generalized atherosclerosis, stroke, and cardiovascular disease. Additionally, there is a tendency toward more accidents from a loss of balance and more severe trauma resulting from accidents when they do occur. Shortness of breath, lack of energy, and depression also are all more likely among the obese.

In a study of 268 volunteers over the age of 60 who lived in central North Carolina, Dr. Erdman Palmore reported that overweight was an excellent predictor of longevity. Not only did more overweight people die, the quality of their lives was poorer. The overweight group had almost three times as many members who spent more than two weeks a year in bed with illness, and 14 percent more were hospitalized. Twenty-one percent more of the overweight individuals reported that their health was bad. The moral: overweight shortens life and adds misery to living.

CALORIC RESTRICTION—REMARKABLE FOR RATS AND BENEFICIAL FOR HUMANS

The first dramatic evidence that the life span of mammals was not immutably fixed by their genes was provided less than fifty years ago by Dr. Clive McCay. While human beings have for centuries dreamed of extending the life span and have invented all kinds of elixirs and potions to recapture youth, modern biologists have become more and more skeptical about the possibility of exceeding the genetic upper limit. Thus, Dr. McCay's discovery—that the life span of rats could be significantly extended by dietary means—was extraordinary. It reopened the possibility that life could be extended at a time when many scientists had reluctantly decided that extension of the life span was not feasible.

The experiment showed that rats fed calorically restricted diets (which were sufficient in nutrients) had their physical growth permanently stunted, in that none attained the weight of rats allowed free access to food. The main effect of this growth retardation appeared to be the maintenance of a "youthful" appearance and the production of a significant delay in the development of diseases which normally kill rats. These results have been confirmed and extended in a number of laboratories with many strains of rodents. It appears that the effect of food restriction operates at the early end of the life span, prolonging "childhood." Calorie-restricted rats do not attain sexual maturity as long as they are underfed. McCay described his underfed rats as remaining active and appearing young whatever their chronological ages. These rats were extremely alert and had a much slower pulse rate than normal.

While the effect of avoiding obesity in man is similar to the effect in rats, it has not been demonstrated that severe caloric restriction in childhood extends life span in humans. Victims of starvation diets appear to age prematurely rather then to retain youthful appearance and vigor. Of course, starvation is different from caloric restriction inasmuch as its victims get less vitamins and nutrients as well as fewer calories. Nevertheless, even various strains of mice have different reactions to food restriction, and humans who are genetically far more diverse would undoubtedly respond very differently to caloric restriction in early life. Hence, we know far too little about the effects of diet on longevity to recommend radical dietary alteration in human children. Nevertheless, the evidence indicates that teaching children moderate dietary habits will make them healthier and will lengthen their lives.

While scientists are not free to undertake radical dietary experiments in the general human population, they are free to experiment on themselves. This tactic was taken by Dr. Frederick Hoelzel who influenced the research ideas of Dr. Clive McCay. In the 1920's Hoelzel was already convinced that Americans were shortening their lives by overeating. He saw a problem in convincing his fellow countrymen to cut down, however, because of the hunger pains and lack of energy experienced when dieting by those who were used to overeating. Hoelzel carried out a number of experiments to see if something inert could be added to the diet to give people a feeling of being full. According to Dr. Comfort, Hoelzel said, "I had no difficulty in swallowing moist sea sand seasoned with salt. The swallowing of about four ounces of sand made me feel as if I had eaten a meal. In fact it made me feel for a time as if I had eaten too much. . . . The sand proved too heavy and irritating for repeated use." Apparently Dr. Hoelzel also experimented with glass balls which had similar drawbacks. He finally settled for a filler of cellulose and psyllium seed, and this product is still used in some contemporary reducing treatments.

If Dr. Hoelzel was on the right track in the 1920's in assuming that overeating was life-shortening, the case is even more clear today when half of all deaths in the United States result from coronary heart disease. We have already discussed the significance of elevated serum cholesterol levels as a risk factor in heart disease, and levels of serum cholesterol rise and fall in direct proportion to changes in body weight. Heart disease and stroke both increase dramatically with increasing degrees of overweight. For example, an increase of no more than 50 percent over ideal weight increases the risk for heart disease and stroke by 100 percent in men and by more than 100 percent in women. Diseases of the arteries are also increased in overweight individuals, undoubtedly due to the fact that obesity is related to high blood pressure as well as high cholesterol levels. Diabetes, which also involves high serum cholesterol levels, is another concomitant of obesity. A recent survey reported 31 studies from all parts of the world which showed a positive correlation between overweight and hypertension, and more importantly, there were 19 studies which showed that blood pressure was reduced when excess weight was lost. Losing weight clearly reverses the risk factor of obesity.

A recent study by Dr. J. M. Olefsky and his associates illustrates the effectiveness of weight loss on reversing the life-shortening effects of obesity. He studied men and women who were mildly overweight and engaged them in a program to lose weight. The average weight loss was 24 pounds, a loss attainable by most without a great deal of sacrifice. This modest weight loss had profound metabolic consequences. Among the positive results, cholesterol levels fell from 282 mg/dl—far above the 250 mg danger level—to 223 mg, thus approaching the safe 200 mg. level. Moderate changes in body weight and nutrition led to dramatic changes in risk factors for heart disease. Such data indicate that we do not have to undertake Herculean measures to extend our life expectancy, that simply losing 20 pounds can change many of us from high risk individuals to people safe from the dangers leading to major causes of death.

In addition to reducing risk factors, caloric restriction leading to weight reduction can reduce mortality rates even in groups of older individuals. In an old age home in Madrid a three-year study of dietary restriction was carried out on a group of 120 men and women over the age of 65. Half of the group served as control subjects and received the normal institutional diet which included 2,300 calories a day compromised of 50 grams of protein and 40 grams of fat. The same diet was fed to the sixty experimental subjects on even days of the month, and on the odd days they ate one liter of milk and 500 grams of fresh fruit (885 calories, 36 grams of protein, 40 grams of fat). Over the three-year period of the study, six of the experimental and thirteen of the control subjects died. Thus, the mortality rate was more than twice as high for those on the higher-calorie diet. Members of the low-calorie diet group spent a total of 123 days in the infirmary, while control group members spent a total of 219 days there. The causes of death and diagnoses of illness showed a preponderance of cardiovascular disease in both groups, but the results suggest that the incidence of cardiovascular disease was significantly less in those individuals who consumed fewer calories.

Such results suggest that it is never too late to control our diet and lose weight. Numerous books with diets are on the market to help us do this, and weight reducing clinics and weight-losing groups abound. While fad diets and quick weight loss methods do us more harm than good, gradual weight loss undertaken with the supervision (and blessing) of a physician will set many of us on a more direct path toward living to be 100. Hence, if you have not been able to motivate yourself to lose weight just to make yourself more attractive, lose weight to save your life.

THE ROLE OF NUTRITION IN LONGEVITY

Because humans are genetically diverse, there is no one diet which can be prescribed which would add years to the life of every individual. Indeed, we hear far too much about various nutrients which supposedly *add* years to our lives. We are bombarded with advertisements and magazine articles touting various approaches, and the perspective on what constitutes the "proper" diet can become very clouded in our minds. Hardly a week passes without an article or headline on nutrition and diet in newspapers and magazines. Such a preoccupation with this topic has led many to devise "get-rich-quick" schemes, and fads, faddists, and charlatans in the nutrition industry abound.

The plain fact is that most of our knowledge of the nutritional requirements of man has been derived from the work on experimental animals, particularly the white rat. We have already seen one example, radical caloric restriction, which in the white rat produced dramatic increases in longevity, while in the human would probably produce premature aging. Humans are far more genetically diverse than inbred strains of laboratory animals, and animals have different nutritional requirements from humans. And, since we cannot experiment with humans as we can with rats, our knowledge about optimal diet and nutrition in humans must come primarily from observational studies of various groups who are either long- or short-lived, and from a few experimental studies in which we manipulate nutritional parameters which we are pretty sure will neither negatively nor drastically affect the participants. In the case of the observational studies, we can never be sure that the short- and long-lived groups differ on the basis of their dietary practices, or if their genes, or environment, or lifestyles cause the differences. In the case of the experiments, because we cannot radically alter the diet, the rsults we get are usually not terribly dramatic.

In the light of these limitations on research on nutrition and longevity, it is remarkable that we have as much information as we do. At the present time we know more about what to avoid in terms of diet than what has beneficial effects. For example, studies of longevous peoples around the world have led us to believe that the avoidance of excessive calories is critical in longevity. In such a study, Alexander Leaf reported that in addition to genetic and lifestyle factors which set many long-lived groups of people apart from shorter-lived Americans, their caloric consumption throughout their lives is lower than consumption in the United States (the American's average daily intake is estimated to be 3,300 calories). Contrasted to the more than 3,000 calories consumed each day by Americans is the 1200-calorie-a-day diet of the people of Vilcabamba, a region in the Andes Mountains in Ecuador. In this underdeveloped region where modern medical technology is unavailable, 16.4 percent of the people are over 65 years of age. Throughout their lives they eat a diet low in animal protein and fat which consists primarily of carbohydrate. The Hunza people living in an isolated region in Pakistan are another longevous people who eat most of their calories in carbohydrates and avoid meat and dairy products. Their average caloric intake is around 1925 calories per day. In the Soviet Republic of Abkhasia which lies between the northeast shores of the Black Sea and the main range of the Caucasus Mountains, live another group of people known for unusually long life and good health. These people live on 1700 to 1900 calories a day with a diet high in dairy products and protein, but relatively low in fat. While the diets of these three groups of longevous people vary greatly in the foods consumed, a common feature is a caloric content of less than 2,000 and a relatively low level of fat.

Another series of associations which have been made in studies of human nutrition are the relationships between diet and various diseases. By studying the diets of individuals with these ailments and by altering their diets, it has been possible to identify certain types of foods which are associated with the diseases.

Diabetes

There are two general types of diabetes. One type, occurring in childhood, is called juvenile-onset diabetes and requires treatment with insulin. The more common form of the disease, maturity-onset diabetes, usually occurs in middle age. It is less severe and can generally be controlled by diet and exercise. Maturity-onset diabetes is the form which is discussed here.

With increasing age all of us are more prone to be diabetic because with age there is an impaired ability for the body to use glucose or blood sugar. By middle age the ability of an individual to metabolize excess glucose in the blood is 75 percent as efficient as that ability in a young person. In old age this system is only 50 percent as effective. Death rate due to diabetes increases rapidly with age, showing a dramatic upswing in the 40's for blacks and in the 50's for whites. The incidence of diabetes is much greater in the black than in the white population, and while a genetic factor cannot be ruled out (since diabetes runs in families), economic and dietary differences are considered to be the primary reason for the different incidence of diabetes in American racial groups.

That diet and lifestyle are more important than genes in diabetes was illustrated in a study of Yemenite Jews who immigrated to Israel. The incidence of diabetes of the new arrivals was 0.05 percent, while in Yemenite Jews who had been living in Israel for longer than ten years the incidence was ten times greater.

Studies of aboriginal societies have indicated the same tenfold increase in the rate of diabetes when dietary habits have changed from primitive to a more refined, westernized-type of diet. Thus, diabetes is another disease associated with modernization. At the turn of the century it was the 27th cause of death in the United States, while it was recently ranked fourth. Since most diabetics die of premature cardiovascular disease, it may be even more prevalent as a cause of death than is reported.

Specific nutrients appear to be important in the development of diabetes. Dr. W. O. Caster, Professor of Nutrition at the University of Georgia, recently found that caproic acid which is present in butterfat and coconut oil produces diabetic symptoms in experimental animals. In searching for commercially-available foods that might provide elevated levels of caproic acid and its derivatives, he found that corn grits and chicken skin were particularly effective in reducing rats' ability to metabloize blood sugar. Such a diet has similarities to the grits-greens-fatback diet characteristic of the poor and black of the Southeastern United States, and it is precisely this population group which shows a marked increase in the incidence of diabetes. Dr. Caster also suggested that potato chips and other sources of heated, oxidized fats may also affect glucose tolerance level, while he suspects that vitamin E and other antioxidants may have a beneficial effect in warding off diabetes.

Strong arguments have been made for a diabetes-inducing effect by high intake of sugar and/or refined starch, but there is not general agreement on this fact because obesity and diabetes have been observed in populations which have low sugar consumption. Dietary carbohydrate and crude fiber intake may protect against diabetes, while high fat intake does increase the risk for the disease.

There is little doubt that obesity is a risk factor for maturity-onset diabetes. Seventy-five percent of such diabetic patients are obese at the time of diagnosis, and weight reduction has a very positive effect on the disease. High-fat diets are particularly successful in producing obesity in animals, and since high fat content in the diet appears to be conducive to diabetes, the main type of food to avoid in excess to prevent this disease appears to be fat. Once the disease is diagnosed, diet can be altered to normalize metabolism. The best diet appears to consist of 1,500-2,000 calories per day with 25-35 percent of the calories comprised of fat, 20 percent protein, and the remainder in carbohydrates. Such a diet begins to approximate the lifetime diet of the longevous peoples described previously, although it still exceeds these diets in protein and particularly in fat content. In laboratory animals bred to have diabetes, overfeeding caused the animals to die prematurely, while caloric restriction delayed or prevented the onset of the disease and normalized the life span. Thus, there is evidence in human and in experimental animal studies indicating that diet dramatically affects the likelihood of the development of maturity-onset diabetes, and that dietary intervention can have beneficial results.

Coronary Heart Disease

The relationship between risk factors and coronary heart disease has been discussed in Chapter 5, along with the interventions, including nutritional interventions, which can reduce the risk. Thus, only a few additional points about nutrition and heart disease need be added here.

The nutritionist, Dr. W. O. Caster, recently stated that with regard to cardiovascular disease it would be prudent for the entire middle-aged population in this country to change the nature of the fat in its diet. Much of the saturated animal fat should be replaced with polyunsaturated vegetable oils. Indeed, this prescription should not be limited to the middle-aged members of our society who are most at risk for heart disease. Proper nutritional patterns should be laid down early in life and carried out through old age. No age group should be exempted from Dr. Caster's proposed regimen.

As has been noted, the correlation between cholesterol intake and cardiovascular mortality is high. However, other characteristics of the diet of developed countries are also strongly implicated. In one study, correlations were compiled between various foods and the mortality rate for coronary heart disease. It was found that animal protein, meat, total fat, egg and sugar consumption, and total calories were very strongly related to heart disease. Americans also use too much salt, which has been directly related to high blood pressure, as has been caffeine which has a definite effect on the cardiovascular system. Individuals who consume more of these foods are found to have a much greater probability of dying of a heart attack. Other foods, such as fish, vegetable fat, and vegetables, appear to have no relationship with heart attacks, while starch and vegetable protein are eaten by people who do not have cardiovascular problems. The message is clear. To avoid heart attacks we must eat less red meat, eggs, and sugar, while increasing our consumption of vegetables, whole grains, and fish.

Cancer

The information available on nutritional relationships to cancer is so spotty at the present time that it appears premature to identify foods which may be involved with certain kinds of cancer. Cross-cultural studies suggest that certain diets high in cereal content preclude individuals to stomach cancer, and most of the observed relationships between cancer and diet involve various parts of the digestive system and the genitals. High fat diets have been associated with increased incidence of cancer, and given the risk such diets create for coronary heart disease and diabetes, it is safe to say that such diets should be avoided. Other potent carcinogens which should be mentioned are nitrosamines which are associated with bacon and preserved meat products. They have been shown to be capable of inducing cancer in many different parts of the body. Food additives such as some red dyes have also been implicated in the cause of cancer.

THE LOW-FAT, LOW-CHOLESTEROL DIET: A LIFESAVER

Dramatic evidence has been presented relating obesity and diet to the major killing diseases in our country. The evidence that a diet high in saturated fats leads to cardiovascular disease is substantial. There is no longer any question that obesity leads to hypertension and that weight loss lowers blood pressure. The relationship between obesity, high fat intake, and diabetes is also very clear, and high fat diets have also been associated with increased incidence of cancer. Overeating in childhood is particularly unfortunate because it sets a pattern more difficult to break and shortens life expectancy. A lifelong diet excessive in calories, in saturated fat, and in refined sugars leads to premature aging and death. One must have a very strong genetic predisposition for long life to survive 100 years eating this kind of diet, and few of us Americans do.

A low-fat, low-cholesterol dietary program can extend your life and the lives of your family. The following outline modified from Dr. Lester Morrison's *Low Fat Way of Health and Longer Life* (Prentice-Hall) will give you some idea of the kinds of foods to eat and what to avoid. Sample menus and an extended discussion of the benefits of this approach are provided by Dr. Morrison in his book and in a number of other cookbooks and books on nutrition and healthful living (some of which are listed in the Appendix).

FOOD TO BE ENJOYED

Soups: The kind of soups to emphasize are bouillons and consommés since they are high in nutrition, filling, and low in calories and fats. They can be served warmed or chilled. Use fat-free vegetable soups, vegetable broths, and soups prepared with skimmed milk. *It is imperative to remove all visible fat and grease from the soup.* Dry soup mixes are quite low in fat, as are vegetable and vegetable-beef canned soups.

Meats: Beef, veal, and lamb are naturally high in both visible and "invisible" fat and cholesterol. However, they are good sources of protein and can be prepared in a manner which is healthful. In this diet, much of the fat allowance is contained in these meats. When the meat is still raw, visible fat must be carefully trimmed off, and during the cooking the fat must be drained. An ideal way of removing most of the fat content is to partially cook the meat, refrigerate the meat and broth, and remove the layer of grease that hardens and floats to the top. Buy lean meats and do not fry them.

Among meats, pork cuts of all kinds, including bacon and ham, are highest in fat and cholesterol content, and they should be eaten only occasionally. This is also true of sausages, brains, sweetbreads, and kidneys.

It is best to avoid gravies, and if they are prepared, great pains should be taken to separate out the fat. Low-fat cookbooks have recipes for preparing gravy in this manner. Garnishes such as watercress, parsley, celery, carrots, radishes, pimento, pickles, paprika, green peppers, cucumbers, mushrooms, and onions can be used to flavor meats instead of using gravy. Seasonings such as garlic, cloves, thyme, marjoram, basil, oregano, bay, and peppermint, and relishes such as mint jelly, mint sauce, chili, catsup, cranberry jelly, chutney are also helpful.

Fish: Excellent low-fat eating is provided by fish. Fish especially low in fat are perch, haddock, flounder, sturgeon, smelts, and scallops. Brook trout, porgy, cod, and croakers are somewhat higher in fat content, but compared to meats, these fish are still very low-fat foods. Canned fish such as tuna when packed in water, is also low in fat. Shellfish such as shrimp, lobster, clams, mussels, and crab should be avoided due to its high cholesterol content.

Poultry: Protein is provided by chicken and turkey which have little fat or cholesterol if they are lean. Dark meat is higher in fat than white meat, and skin and giblets should be avoided because of their high fat content. Guinea hen and squab are comparatively low in fat, while duck and goose are extremely high.

Eggs: The whites of eggs are high in protein and they may be eaten with no problem. Egg yolk contains a high concentration of cholesterol and should be avoided. Egg substitutes on the market provide a simulation of whole egg without the cholesterol.

Milk and Milk Products: Non-fat or skim milk is acceptable, and a pint or more daily is recommended. Buttermilk and low-fat yogurt are also okay.

Cheeses: Butterfat content in cheese is high, so the majority of them should be avoided. Cottage cheese made from non-fat milk is an exception (but be sure to avoid creamed cottage cheese). Ricotta cheese and jack cheese made from skim milk or whey can also be safely eaten on this diet.

Vegetables: Almost no fat or cholesterol is contained in vegetables. The use of butter or other fats in the preparation of vegetables must be avoided, and herbs and seasonings or bouillon should be substituted in preparation and serving. Better yet, serve vegetables raw to obtain maximum vitamin and mineral content.

Fruits: Little fat and no cholesterol is contained in fruits. The only exceptions are avocado and coconut which are both very high in fat content. Avoid them. Other fruits can be enjoyed throughout the day, and they are particularly useful as desserts.

Salads and Salad Dressings: Raw vegetables are best, but gelatin and aspic salads are also acceptable. Salad dressings, when used, should be low in fat content. The best are prepared at home, and recipes can be found in low-fat cookbooks.

Cereals: These products are free of fat and are nutritious and energy producing. All cooked or dry cereals are good sources of carbohydrates. They should be served with non-fat milk and a minimal amount of sugar. Of course, sugar-coated cereals are best avoided.

Breads: Another source of carbohydrate is bread. Whole wheat bread is the more nutritious form. Yeast loaf bread, sweet rolls, rolls, muffins, buns, and coffee cake should be eaten only occasionally because of their high calorie content and because they typically contain lard, butter, or egg yolk.

Desserts: The best dessert is fruit. Most other sweet foods are high in calories, although some, such as jam, jelly, marmalade, honey, molasses, maple syrup, hard candies, and candies without nuts, creams, or chocolate are fat-free. Regardless of the fat-free nature of these sweets, however, they are best avoided or eaten only occasionally.

Beverages: Tea, coffee, coffee substitutes, skim or fat-free milk, non-fat milk, cocoa, skim milk powder shakes, and egg white eggnogs are all free of fat. Fruit and vegetable juices are also good. Carbonated drinks such as ginger ale, Coco-Cola, 7-Up and others are free of fat, but high in calories. Sugar-free carbonated drinks avoid this problem, but some question as to the safety of the sweeteners in these beverages has been raised. Of course, water is an important source of liquid in the diet, and drinking 6 to 8 glasses a day reduces the need for other beverages as well as helping to flush fat waste products out of the system.

Foods to Avoid

Soups: All creamed soups, particularly commercially prepared ones, are heavy in fat.

Meats: Sweetbreads, brains, kidneys, caviar, fish roe, and giblets are high in cholesterol and fat content. They should be avoided. Pork and pork products, bacon, and ham should be eaten only occasionally.

Fish: High-fat fish are bass, bluefish, butterfish, deviled crab, eel, herring, mackerel, scalloped or fried oysters, pompano, salmon, sardines, shad, and trout. High-cholesterol fish are clams, crab, lobster, mussels, and shrimp.

Poultry: Duck and goose should be avoided unless prepared in a fat-free manner.

Dairy Products: Eliminate from the diet whole milk, cream, butter, and cheeses such as American, cheddar, Swiss, cream, creamed cottage, cheese spreads, Gruyere, Edam, Limberger, Liederkranz, Parmesan, Roquefort, and yogurt made from whole milk.

Eggs: Egg yolks may be the single most potent source of cholesterol in the American diet, and they are to be avoided.

Breads: Hot breads, pancakes, waffles, coffee cakes, muffins, buns, doughnuts, Danish pastry, and sweet rolls are high in calories and contain lard, butter, or egg yolk. If you simply must have such breads, find fat-free recipes for them in low-fat cookbooks and bake them at home.

Desserts: Anything made with butter, egg yolks, or cream such as pie, cake, pastry, cookies, custard, eclairs, gingerbread, shortcake, and pudding should be eliminated from the diet. Ice cream, parfaits, and frozen creams have far too much fat and cholesterol to be healthful.

Miscellaneous Foods: Avocados, coconuts, nuts, chocolate, cocoa, and fat in salad dressings, gravies, and sauces should be avoided. Do not cook with animal fats including lard and suet. If you cook with fats at all, substitute vegetable fats. Frying must be completely eliminated in the preparation of foods. Alcohol has no fat content, but drinking should be moderate as alcohol is high in calories.

DO VITAMINS AFFECT LONGEVITY?

Perhaps the favorite type of nutrient to be advocated by various individuals and groups is the vitamin. Vitamins may also be the easiest dietary alteration to advocate because they can be ingested without modifying other aspects of our eating habits. It would be wonderful, indeed, if we could find some little pill which we could swallow painlessly each day and which would make us healthier and more longevous. Unfortunately, while several vitamins may have moderately beneficial effects, none so far has been found which has miraculous properties.

One of the problems which clouds the issue of whether benneficial effects are derived from certain vitamins is the "placebo" effect. Any change in a person's life, which he or she perceives as potentially helpful, may lead the person to feel better, whether or not the treatment itself is effective. This has clearly been the case with vitamin B_{12} injections. No statistics are available on the number of people (usually older people) who routinely receive such therapy, and whether an improvement in the overall well-being of individuals results from such supplementation is still open to question. Nevertheless, many who have received the treatment swear by it. It is true that vitamin B_{12} levels decline with age, even in very healthy individuals, so there is some rationale for the injections. It is not certain, however, that the older system can assimilate the injected vitamin and profit from it. Thus, at the present time only the psychological benefits of B_{12} injections have been documented. Since the only negative factor is the expense of the shot, who is to deny such therapy to those older people who maintain that they secure great benefits and who can afford it? Additional research may even prove that their enthusiasm has been justified.

In an article on the possible role of vitamins in the aging process, Dr. Olaf Mickelsen of Michigan State University was only willing to endorse one vitamin as possibly having positive effects on health and longevity. This vitamin is vitamin C. The effects of this vitamin appear to have been studied more extensively than any other. Dr. Mickelsen concluded that the results of a number of studies indicate that a higher than normal intake of vitamin C reduces the aches and pains to which older people are prone, lowers mortality when the aged are ill, and increases their longevity. It appears that generally there is a low vitamin C content in the diets of older people, and supplements ranging from 50 to 200 mg. daily do have beneficial effects. Since excess vitamin C is excreted rather than retained in the body, it seems safe to recommend a daily vitamin C supplement of 100-200 mg. as a protection against the deleterious effects of excessively low levels of this vitamin.

The vitamin which has probably received the most attention recently with regard to aging and longevity is vitamin E. Controlled human studies on this vitamin have not appeared as they have on vitamin C, so the available data are much more inferential, drawn from animal work and work with cells in tissue culture. If one is to believe the cellular work, vitamin E is indeed beneficial. It appears to reduce build up of fats and other deleterious substances associated with aging in the body. In experiments with cell cultures, vitamin E doubled the number of times the cells could normally divide, thus doubling the life span of the tissue culture. In aging experimental animals, vitamin E has been observed to prevent the buildup of deleterious substances. However, there is no clear evidence that taking the antitoxant vitamin E improves human longevity. Indeed, amounts taken by vitamin enthusiasts which may exceed one gram a day could even be harmful. One hundred units of vitamin E a day most probably will not harm us, and could possibly serve to keep our veins and arteries freer from the build-up of fatty deposits. Under no circumstances, however, should we believe that taking vitamin E can compensate for our high-fat American diet. The best preventative medicine is to change the diet. *In addition,* we may decide to take the added precaution of ingesting some vitamin E.

7.
Warning:
Smoking is Hazardous
to Your Health

&➤The one thing which you can do to extend your life expectancy most is to stop smoking. In fact, there is nothing subtracting more years from your life than smoking two packs of cigarettes a day. If you are not a smoker, then you have already saved a number of years of your life. If you are a reformed smoker, you should congratulate yourself for having reduced your risk of a premature death. For at least twenty years there has been little question that smoking is harmful to health. Although powerful lobbyists for cigarette manufacturers, such as The Tobacco Institute, would have you believe that the research has not clearly demonstrated a relationship between cigarette smoking and a number of chronic, life-shortening diseases, these self-serving propagandists are doing you an extreme disservice. Not only does the tar, nicotine, and carbon monoxide from your cigarette pollute your lungs and poison you, the second-hand smoke from your cigarette has deleterious effects on those around you—your friends and your family.

In spite of two decades of warnings about the dangers of smoking and in spite of the numerous negative consequences of smoking felt by smokers, 25 percent of the adult population of Americans still smoke. Indeed, more and more women are adopting the smoking habit, with a host of serious consequences to themselves and their offspring. The first six years of the 1970's have witnessed almost a doubling of the number of female smokers in the 12- to 18-year-old category. Since 1930, about the time it became socially acceptable for women to smoke, deaths among women from lung cancer have increased by more than 400 percent. It has been estimated that if all men quit smoking, the eight-year sex difference in longevity would be cut in half. If smoking among women continues to increase, the gap between the sexes in longevity will narrow.

One of the most heartening trends in years is the recently reported statistic that physicians in great numbers are giving up cigarettes. Many lung cancer patients or recent victims of heart attacks undoubtedly found it difficult to follow the advice of their doctor who told them with a cigarette in his mouth that they should quit smoking. Apparently physicians themselves believe the dramatic evidence demonstrating that smoking leads to poor health, and they are taking the responsibility of setting the proper model for their patients.

Why is it that in the face of overwhelming evidence that smoking is dangerous, and in spite of the inconvenience and expense of the habit, we have such a difficult time giving it up? Are there positive benefits to smoking which offset the hazards? Is smoking a hallmark of our contemporary age of stress?

It turns out that smoking has been with us throughout history. There are archeological reports of pipe smoking among the South American Indians in Venezuela 8,000 years ago. There is even a Greek myth about the advent of tobacco on the earth. The story goes that Zeus was banqueting with his gods and goddesses on Mount Olympus, and after the sumptuous meal they began to dance. Vulcan, the god of fire, was urged to dance, but he was ashamed because of his hunchback and his fear of derision. To cover his nervousness and embarrassment he lit his pipe and filled Olympus with a black cloud of foul-smelling smoke. This rude behavior enraged Zeus who cast a thunderbolt at the pipe, smashing it and spreading bits of pipe tobacco all over the world. The tobacco seed took root and grew on the earth, and ever since man has been able to cure it and adopt Vulcan's foul habit.

Dr. Lester Morrison, a California physician who tells the above myth, also noted that the controversy about the dangers of smoking is not a 20th century phenomenon. The same controversy raged 350 years ago. In 1604, the King of England, James I, was anxious to improve the health of his subjects. He consulted with his court physicians, and issued the following proclamation on tobacco: "A custom loathsome to the eye, hateful to the nose, harmful to the brain, dangerous to the lungs, and in the black stinking fumes thereof, nearest resembling the horrible Stygian smoke of the hell pit that is bottomless."[1]

Half a century later the French came to a similar conclusion. Physicians at the Medical School of Paris studied and reported on the effects of tobacco smoking on health and longevity. Their conclusion was that tobacco smoking shortens life. Among the harmful effects of smoking they included: colic, diarrhea, ulcerations of the lungs, asthma, coughs, pains in the heart, undernourishment, and impotence. In the 16th and 17th centuries less benevolent rulers not only warned of the dangers of smoking—they imposed the death penalty for it. Smokers of this period faced a double risk of premature death from smoking. If the tar and nicotine did not kill them, the king's soldiers would. Nevertheless, tobacco smoking flourished, much as it does today under the imposing death sentence it incurs.

There must be powerful benefits and pleasures from smoking for people to risk so much. What are these attributes? Smoking has been incorporated as a part of social life since its existence was first reported. It helps relax people and makes them more sociable. The tradition of smoking the peace pipe among American Indians is a classic example of the hostility-reducing properties of ceremonial smoking. Tobacco has been used in religious ceremonies and on social occasions in a number of different ways. According to Dr. Morrison, it has been smoked, swallowed, chewed, drunk in various concoctions, gargled, sniffed, and licked. Another use for tobacco has been as a health potion. It has been used in enemas and applied to wounds. A more common use of tobacco is to soothe the nerves in times of anxiety and crises. It is often used to relieve pain and shock and can serve as a sedative permitting the smoker to sleep in times of trauma. Pleasure smokers take a cigarette break to relax and enjoy a feeling of light-headedness. The relaxation provided by a cigarette after a meal is one of the hardest things for smokers to give up. Another thing people find positive about smoking is that it creates a habit which provides security. They look forward to their next cigarette as it paces their day. It also provides nervous people with something to do with their hands. Unfortunately, those desiring these simple pleasures provided by cigarettes pay an awesome price. The consequences of smoking are extensive—and they are fatal.

THE DEADLY EFFECTS OF SMOKING

Few people recognize the fact that tobacco is a very potent poison. If you were to eat two or three cigarettes, they would kill you. The reason for this is that nicotine, a major ingredient in tobacco, is poisonous. It affects the brain, the heart, and other vital organs. The amount of nicotine required to kill an adult human is from 60 to 120 milligrams. You inhale about 2 milligrams of nicotine when you smoke one cigarette, but if you ate it, you would consume 100-200 milligrams. Think of the consequences if your baby found your pack of cigarettes and ate even half a cigarette. There are thousands of cases of accidental deaths, suicides, and murders recorded each year by governmental agencies resulting from nicotine poisoning.

Other poisons contained in burning tobacco are arsenic, coal tar, and carbon monoxide. The former contribute to cancer in the mouth, esophagus, and respiratory tract, while carbon monoxide leads to oxygen deprivation causing premature aging of tissue such as the skin.

All kinds of chronic health problems are associated with cigarette smoking, and the more cigarettes smoked per day, the greater the incidence of disease. The results of a Public Health service survey in the United States between the years of 1964 and 1965 make it is clear that smoking and chronic health conditions go hand in hand. Smoking appears to affect the health of the young more than the health of the old, with non-smokers in the younger age groups recording a lower incidence of chronic disease than do smokers, while chronic disease in old non-smokers is almost as high as it is in smokers. This is true primarily because the incidence of chronic disease increases with age. So many of the heavy smokers have died before they reach 65, that they could not be counted in the statistics for that age group, and those smokers surviving that long probably have inherited such a strong genetic constitution that they survive in spite of smoking. These old, heavy smokers may be the people who initially had the best chance of reaching the age of 100, but few will make it because they cut off many of those extra years gained from heredity by smoking. If you are inclined to gamble with smoking in the hope that you are one of those rare individuals who is extremely well-endowed genetically, don't. The chances are very small that you are one of the few to escape the hazards of smoking—and in the end, no one escapes. You could live even longer and with better health if you quit.

There is a wide range of negative effects resulting from smoking. The three major chronic diseases linked to tobacco are lung cancer, chronic bronchitis, and coronary heart disease. The risk for these diseases is considerably less for pipe and cigar smokers than for cigarette smokers, but cancers of the mouth, larynx, and esophagus are more frequent in all types of smokers than in non-smokers. Smoking in women leads to smaller birth weight of their infants and increased risk of spontaneous abortion, stillbirth, and death during the first days of life. Less serious consequences include yellow teeth, foul breath, and wrinkled skin.

HOW SMOKING AFFECTS THE BODY

The Lungs

According to Dr. T. M. Perry—and undisputed among epidemiologists—is that fact that cancer of the lung and bronchus is the chief "new disease" among the various types of cancer. Prior to 1930 it was so infrequently diagnosed on death certificates that it was not coded as a separate item. It was lumped into the category of "other neoplasms." Classic pathology textbooks used in medical school in the 1920's identified cancer of the lung as being responsible for 1 to 2 percent of all cancers. In the 1970's, cancer of the lung accounts for 20 percent of the deaths resulting from cancer. Dr. Perry cites increased cigarette smoking as the major factor in this trend.[2] The American Cancer Society reported that moderate cigarette smokers (10 to 15 cigarettes per day) have *five times* as many lung cancers as non-smokers. Heavy cigarette smokers (16 to 25 cigarettes per day) have *fifteen times* as many lung cancers as non-smokers, and excessively heavy cigarette smokers (25 to 50 cigarettes per day) have *twenty-five times* as many lung cancers as non-smokers.

The cancer-producing substances in cigarettes seem to be the coal tars released in the burning cigarette. About 50 percent of the solid particles inhaled in tobacco smoke are deposited in the bronchial tubes, and included in this deposit are nicotine, coal tars, and many other products. These particles act as irritants. Listen to the chronic cough and speaking voice of heavy, long-time smokers. To test the effect yourself, all you have to do is check your wind after having a few cigarettes. Better yet, compare your breathing after climbing several flights of stairs before and after you quit smoking.

Since pipe and cigar smokers do not ordinarily inhale, the incidence of lung cancer from smoking pipes and cigars is very much lower than the incidence from smoking cigarettes. Excessively heavy pipe and cigar smokers (more than 50 grams of pipe tobacco or 10 to 15 cigars per day) have an increased incidence of cancer of the lips, mouth, tongue, and gums.

The Heart and Arteries

Just as smokers can feel the effect of smoking on their breathing, they can feel it affecting their hearts. Toxic effects on the heart are noticed when the patient experiences the heart skipping several beats or palpitating. Heart abnormalities due to smoking are often manifested as dizziness, shortness of breath, headaches (due to increases in blood pressure, or pains and distress over the chest. Tobacco produces pain and stress on the heart when it is already damaged or weakened by some other condition, particularly coronary atherosclerosis. Tobacco smoking causes constriction of the coronary arteries which can do more damage to the heart.

Blood pressure can be dramatically elevated by smoking. Some research has shown a 40 mm/Hg rise in systolic blood pressure resulting from smoking. This great increase is enough to put a person at low-risk for blood pressure (systolic pressure of 125 mm/Hg) into the high risk category 165 mm/Hg). In patients with high blood pressure who are already at risk for heart attack, smoking in moderate to heavy amounts has a strong tendency to elevate blood pressure by even more than 40 mm/Hg. Anyone with known heart disease or high blood pressure who continues to smoke might as well play with a loaded gun.

Smoking has a pronounced effect on the blood vessels in all parts of the body. Vessels constrict under the influence of tobacco, thus producing poorer circulation. Poor circulation in the hands, legs, and feet is characteristic of heavy smokers. Indeed, nicotine is one of the worst poisons to the blood vessels. Disease such as Buerger's disease which is a condition in which blood vessels, particularly vessels in the legs, are obliterated are associated with smoking. Victims of this disease often must have a leg amputated because gangrene results from the poor circulation.

A grotesque story of a patient with Buerger's disease is told by Dr. Morrison, who as part of his medical training had to be exposed to those suffering from this disease. He reacted with horror to the roomful of amputees, many of whom had lost one or two legs from gangrene. One man made a particularly startling impression on the doctor. This man had lost both legs and still could not stop smoking. At the time of Dr. Morrison's visit he was about to lose an arm. In the face of losing all of his limbs the man insisted that he would rather die than give up smoking. It was not long after that that the smoking finally killed him. Buerger's disease is rare, but hundreds of thousands of Americans make the same decision made by this man, and are killed by cancer or heart disease as a result of their refusal to give up cigarette smoking.

Raynaud's syndrome is also associated with excessive smoking. With this disease the small blood vessels in the hands, feet, nose, cheek, and ears constrict in an irregular fashion causing blanching of the skin and pain upon exposure to cold, anxiety, fatigue, physical pressure or shock. Patients suffering from atherosclerosis also exacerbate their disease by smoking as they increase the constriction of the vessels already present as a result of the condition.

The Digestive Tract

The view that most smokers hold is that smoking aids their digestion. They believe this because they relax and feel better after a meal if they smoke. These pleasant feelings are misleading, because tobacco is an irritant to all parts of the digestive system. The lines and cracks developing in the tongue as a result of smoking place it in a condition prone to cancer, and this cancer may spread to the mouth and to other parts of the digestive tract. Gastritis, or local inflammation of the stomach, if often produced by smoking because nicotine is absorbed into the saliva and carried to the stomach. Stomach ulcers are always aggravated by smoking, and ulcer patients are well-advised to quit. Thus, the toxins in tobacco penetrate even those parts of the body to which the smoke does not travel. They travel in the blood and in the saliva, and poison parts of the body seemingly protected from the damaging effects.

The Skin

The visible damage of smoking—the damage done to the skin—has been studied by Dr. Harry Daniell of California. While this damage is not hazardous to physical health, it dramatically affects appearance, which may in turn affect mental health. Over a one-year period, Dr. Daniell observed a large number of patients ranging in age from 30 to 70 years. He examined them clinically and recorded a wrinkle score on the basis of wrinkles in the left crow's foot area around the eye. In each age group the most heavily wrinkled people were smokers, and over the period of the study, smokers developed more wrinkles than non-smokers. This effect occurred in both men and women. Smokers in the 40- to 49-year-old group were as prominently wrinkled as non-smokers twenty years their senior. Thus, while smokers may never live to be 100, they may look 100 years old before they die.

HOW TO QUIT SMOKING

The pleasant sensations associated with smoking and the physical addiction some people develop to it make abandoning the habit very difficult. Few smokers, however, develop so severe an addiction that, given enough incentive, they can't quit or cut down without destroying the meaning of their life.

There are a number of ways to improve your health by reducing your reliance on tobacco. One way to begin is to cut down on the number of cigarettes you smoke each day. Eliminating one or two cigarettes per day is the easiest way for some people to reduce their smoking habit. Smoking cigarettes with lower tar and nicotine levels and stronger filters helps. Eventually, when you have cut down to five or six cigarettes a day, you may be at a point where you can quit entirely. That is by far the most healthy solution.

Switching to a pipe is another means of continuing a tobacco habit while reducing the health hazards. Unfortunately, it is socially less acceptable for women to smoke pipes than for men. Even for women, however, attractive pipes are being made, and appearance-conscious women may find lighting up a pipe less unattractive than the wrinkles they will surely get if they continue smoking.

Chewing gum and hard candies are a means some people use to substitute for their oral craving for cigarettes. Sucking on sugar-free gum or candy eliminates the calorie and cavity risk of eating a lot of sweets.

Apart from substitutes, there are behavior modification techniques used in anti-smoking clinics to help people quit. Some find that hypnosis or therapy is useful, while others have deconditioned themselves by painting silver nitrate on the tip of their tongues to make the cigarettes taste bitter. Before undertaking this route, consult your physicial so that you don't poison yourself or do undue damage to your tongue.

The best way to stop smoking is to exert your will power and simply quit. President Eisenhower exemplified this method after he had a heart attack. He was quoted at a news conference as stating that the only way he knew to quit smoking was just to stop. Before you have a heart attack or develop symptoms of lung cancer, exert pressure on yourself and quit.

8.
The Uses and Abuses
of Alcohol

ɛ॰The effect of alcohol on health and longevity are quite different from those of cigarette smoking. It is clear that smoking a few cigarettes is bad for you, a few more are worse, and a lot are disastrous for your health. However, there is no such linear relationship between alcohol and longevity. A moderate amount of alcohol does not appear to harm you—in fact, it may even have beneficial effects. On the other hand, people who absolutely abstain from drinking are shown to have slightly shorter life expectancies, and people who over-indulge cut short their lives by a number of years. There seems to be a threshold level for the body's tolerance for alcohol, and amounts below this threshold (two drinks per day or less for most people) have no deleterious effect, while amounts exceeding the threshold (three or more drinks per day) do irreversible damage.

The Department of Health, Education, and Welfare recently releaesd a report, which suggested that alcoholism costs the nation $25 billion a year. There was absolutely no question from the statistics presented that excess alcohol consumption is associated with tragedy. On the other hand, moderate drinkers were found to live longer than abstainers. "Moderate drinking" in this report was considered to be less than three ounces of whiskey, *or* a half-liter of wine, *or* four glasses of beer per day. The major conclusion of the report was that the wide range of devastating problems associated with the use of alcohol all relate to excess, and not to moderation.

This result reported by the government, that moderate drinkers live longer than abstainers, is not a one-time finding or a fluke result due to some sampling error. It is a result which has been replicated in a number of very large, carefully done studies. The effect is also one which has been present for decades, and it was documented by Dr. Raymond Pearl in his extensive research on longevity in Baltimore early in the twentieth century. In 1924 Dr. Pearl published a study on alcohol and life duration based on his work with over 6,000 adults of all ages belonging to the working class population of Baltimore. From this study he concluded, that "moderate" drinkers, whether males or females, and at all ages from 30 up, have a somewhat *higher* life expectancy than the persons of the same age in the "abstainer" class. The "moderate" category was defined by Dr. Pearl as "one who used alcohol in any form (beer, wine, or spirits), but in small amount at any one time and never enough to become intoxicated." This group lived about a year and a half longer than the people who never used alcohol in any form. The typical extensive shortening of life expectancy associated with heavy drinking was also documented by Pearl. Heavy male drinkers lived five and a half years less than moderate drinkers, and heavy female drinkers lived over thirteen years less than their moderate drinking peers.

The most difficult aspect of the relationship between alcohol and longevity to explain is the fact that abstainers have shorter life expectancies than moderate drinkers. There does not seem to be any research which has been undertaken to addrss this issue, and few are even willing to speculate as to why this finding occurs. Nonetheless, the evidence is clear: teetotalers have shorter life expectancies. By why? One possibility is that income plays a role. Moderate drinking may be more characteristic of people in higher income brackets, and these are the people who have longer life expectancy. There may be no relation between the drinking habits themselves and longevity. It just may be that the people who are more likely to be moderate drinkers are more affluent and more able to ensure their own long life.

Another possible explanation for the relationship between shorter life expectancy and abstinence from alcohol is related to personality. People who live the longest appear to be relaxed, tolerant individuals who take life as it comes. They are flexible and happy and able to adapt to changing circumstances. Perhaps people who have rigid value systems leading them to ban liquor absolutely from their homes or lives are rigid in other ways as well. These people may be more likely to suffer from stress. Their blood pressure may be higher, and their health may be poorer as a result of their tenseness.

A third possibility is that many of the people who are counted as abstainers in the statistics are former alcoholics or individuals who know that alcoholism runs in their families. There appears to be some genetic influence on an individual's tolerance of alcohol and on his or her ability to control drinking. If your parents or grandparents were alcoholics, you have to be more careful about your own drinking habit because you are more likely than most to develop a drinking problem. People who have this genetic weakness for alcoholism may also be less well-endowed genetically for long life. Again, it is not the abstaining that causes the shorter life expectancy, it is a genetic characteristic of the individuals who abstain.

One last possibility is that alcohol taken in moderation actually has beneficial effects, and, in fact, when we examine the effects of alcohol on the body we see that moderate doses do have some positive physiological consequences. Alcohol helps people to relax and to escape stress. It also improves the circulation. Whether this has any consequences for life expectancy is unknown, but it could explain why moderate drinkers live longer than abstainers.

What kind of conclusions can we draw from the speculation presented above? First, we must accept the fact that the relationship between moderate drinking and longer life has not been explained. Just because drinking in moderation and longer life are correlated does not mean that moderate drinking *causes* longer life. Three of the four possible explanations for the relationship presented above involve causes totally unrelated to drinking. Moderate drinkers may be of higher socioeconomic status, they may have less rigid personality structures, or they may be free of genetic weaknesses causing shorter life. Only the fourth alternative suggests that moderate drinking may itself cause benefits which extend life.

The reason for being so careful in interpreting the relationship between moderate drinking and longer life is that we are reluctant to advise people who abstain to start drinking moderately. Those who abstain because they know they cannot tolerate alcohol would suffer disastrous consequences from such advice. Some people simply cannot be moderate drinkers—they either must abstain or become alcoholics. If you are in this category, *don't touch the stuff!* If you have good reasons for not drinking, the present state of our knowledge concerning the relationship between alcohol and longevity is just not sufficient to advise you to drink. The only advice warranted by the data at the present time is that you should avoid being tense and rigid and try to relax. A brisk walk for fifteen minutes can be at least as relaxing as a drink, so there is no reason to resort to alcohol.

For those who are moderate drinkers, the data suggest that there is no reason to change your ways. Other than the extra calories contained in alcohol, there appear to be no negative consequences to having a social drink. Just be careful not to mix drinking with driving, or become too reliant on your cocktail.

PHYSIOLOGICAL EFFECTS OF ALCOHOL

Few substances have as mixed an effect on the body as does alcohol. It has been called both a blessing and a curse, a poison and a food. It is a true mass of contradictions. The majority of Americans (68 percent) drink alcoholic beverages, and most of these people are only occasional or moderate drinkers. However, 12 percent admit that they drink heavily. Figure 5 depicts the drinking habits of Americans. What are these various kinds of drinkers doing to their bodies? Dr. Lester Morrison has described some of the beneficial and injurious effects.

Beneficial Effects

Alcohol has the chemical effect of a depressant. It depresses the higher inhibitory centers of the brain, causing the individual to feel less constrained, more impulsive, and more relaxed. Many of us are amazed by our social *savoir faire* and grace under the influence of alcohol. We feel this way because we are less inhibited. Words flow more easily, and we are willing to be more open and take more risks.

For years many physicians have advised patients to take alcoholic beverages in moderate amounts to relax nervous or high-strung behavior, to calm anxieties, and to aid in sleep. Just the thought of a glass of wine or beer is enough to sedate many people; they relax at the idea of drinking as they anticipate the effect. Alcohol can also be used as an out-and-out sedative, narcotic, or analgesic for the relief of pain, distress, or fatigue. To avoid the toxic effects, however, the amount must be small to moderate.

In compounding prescriptions, alcohol is used extensively. In addition to its properties as a solvent and preserving agent, it serves as a dilator of the blood vessels and is helpful in circulation. This is a particularly good feature in the case of older people. Alcohol also stimulates the appetite, thereby enabling greater quantities of food and drink to be consumed. This is one of the reasons why dieters should avoid the drink before a meal. Their appetitie will be stimulated. Another reason why it is hard to lose weight and drink alcoholic beverages is that alcohol contains a high number of calories, and most mixers we use with it have even more calories. The calories in alcohol are not useful as food because they are burned up or oxidized in the form of heat. In this manner they are known as "empty calories" because they are not processed into body tissue. Another effect of alcohol is as a mild stimulant to the kidneys.

This effect leads to an increased output of urine. Metabolic rate and heart rate are increased moderately by alcohol, although when applied directly to the skin, it has a cooling effect. Alcohol is also used widely as an antiseptic.

FIGURE 5. Distribution of Alcohol Consumption in the United States Based on a National Survey of 2,746 Americans.

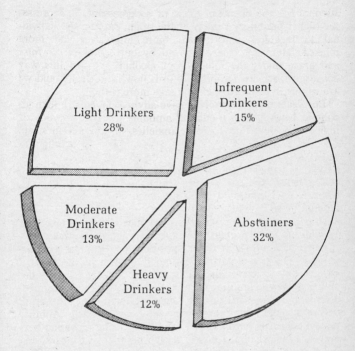

Abstainers—drink less than once a year or not at all; *infrequent drinkers*—drink at least once year, but less than once a month; *light drinkers*—drink at least once a month, but typically only one or two drinks on a single occasion; *moderate drinkers*—drink at least once a month, typically several times, but usually with no more than three or four drinks per occasion; *heavy drinkers*—drink nearly every day with five or more per occasion at least once in awhile, or about once weekly with usually five or more per occasion.

SOURCE: D. Cahalan, I. H. Cisin, and M. Crossley, *A National Study of Drinking Behavior and Attitudes* (New Brunswick, N. J.: Rutgers Center of Alcohol Studies, 1969).

Alcohol has a positive effect on circulation in that it dilates vessels. It has been used by physicians as a vasodilating agent as it increases circulation by widening the peripheral blood vessels on body surfaces and extremities such as the face, hands, legs, and feet. At one time it was also hypothesized that alcohol affected the coronary arteries by dilating them, and that all patients with heart disease should drink alcohol regularly. In fact, many of these patients did experience fewer heart pains when they had drinks before, during, and after meals. More recent evidence, however, indicates that alcohol does not relieve pain in these patients by dilating coronary arteries. The effect occurs because alcohol has an analgesic effect, it desensitizes the patient to pain, and it relaxes the patient so that he or she worries less about the pain. Too much drinking in heart patients is actually dangerous because they may over-exert and strain their hearts in the absence of the warning signal of pain.

Injurious Effects

Excessive drinking has tragic consequences for the individual, his or her family, and society. Crime, suicide, divorce, child abuse, juvenile delinquency, automobile accidents, and economic and industrial losses are all linked with heavy drinking, and, as mentioned previously, alcoholism has been estimated to cost us $25 billion a year. However, the social consequences of heavy drinking and alcoholism are well-known and need not be discussed here. Since our aim is to relate alcohol to longevity, we will concentrate on the physiological effects of excessive drinking.

In addition to the effect of relaxing the mind, alcohol also leads to diminished efficiency, inaccuracy and impairment in judgment, loss of self-reliance, violent behavior, and perhaps diminished resistance to disease in general. Alcohol exerts a paralyzing effect on parts of the brain which control judgment and reason. Double vision, dizziness, nausea, clumsiness, lack of coordination, slowed response time, and loss of self-control are all symptoms of alcoholic excess and reminders that dramatic physiological alterations in our bodies occur as a result of high levels of this substance. While it is harmless in moderate quantities, in excess alcohol is a poison.

An overdose of alcohol, like an overdose of nicotine, can be fatal. Due to wide individual variation, it takes very different amounts of alcohol to kill different people. A fatal dose ranges from one pint to one quart of whiskey, or eight to sixteen ounces of pure alcohol. In children the fatal dose level is much lower. Drivers are considered drunk if their blood contains one-tenth of one percent of alcohol. Death from alcohol can occur indirectly from the crazy stunts or accidents in which intoxicated people are involved, or it can occur as a direct result of too much alcohol which usually kills by paralyzing the respiratory center in the brain. The brain simply forgets to tell the lungs to continue breathing. Thus, alcoholics die at a higher rate from physiological damage directly attributable to the drug, and they also die more frequently than non-alcoholics from violent causes, depression (and suicide), heavy smoking, and malnutrition.

Chronic alcoholism has severe consequences for the brain and nervous system. As a result of vitamin B and C deficiencies caused by excessive alcohol, numerous hemorrhages occur in the brain which result in the death of brain tissue. The brains of alcoholics are particularly susceptible to injuries because the blood vessels are so likely to rupture. Thus, death occurs in alcoholics often as a result of secondary trauma suffered from a blow to the head, such as in the case of a fall or a barroom brawl. Many kinds of paralysis and memory disorders are seen in alcoholics because the parts of the brain controlling these functions have atrophied as a result of the loss of blood supply to these areas. Another frequent nervous system complication of chronic alcoholism results from a lack of vitamin B and ends in destruction in the peripheral nerves. The feet are usually numb, tender, or painful, and the patient may not be able to walk.

Delirium tremens (D.T.) have long been known as a concomittant of alcoholism. The symptoms include confusion, anxiety or terror, auditory and visual hallucinations, and delusions. Patients may be obessed with snakes or other animals (the true "pink elephant" syndrome), or they may feel persecuted by people or voices. Violent tremors and shaking often occur at the same time as the delirious episodes.

Another disease related to chronic alcoholism is Korsakoff's Psychosis. Basically this disease involves the loss of recent memory on the part of the patient. To cover this total inability to remember events which have just occurred, the patient makes up fabulous stories. Since the patient is convinced that the stories are true, many visitors are fooled and amazed by Korsakoff patients. If you were to visit an individual in this condition, he might be very friendly and fascinating, spinning incredible tales about his travels or experiences. You might spend an hour or more talking wh him, and then have to leave the room for a minute. When you returned, the patient would not recognize you and have no memory of your interaction. Truly, for these patients, each day is a bright new day. The recent past in their minds is totally gone.

Cirrhosis of the liver occurs as a consequence of heavy drinking. It is basically a nutritional disease, resulting from inadequate and improper diet in conjunction with excessive drinking. The liver is usually swollen and enlarged at first, but later it shrinks and becomes atrophied. The symptoms of the disease are nervousness, fatigue, dyspepsia, vomiting and passage of blood, and chest and abdominal pains and swelling. The final symptoms are jaundice and coma, and the consequence of cirrhosis of the liver is death. Caught before the final stages, cirrhosis patients will survive—if they can be induced to quit drinking alcoholic beverages completely. Alcoholics Anonymous can be a tremendous help to people in this condition, while psychiatric care may or may not be beneficial. Special diets have also been shown to be effective in treating this disease, but the most important condition appears to be that the patient swears off alcohol of any kind.

There is absolutely no question that excessive alcoholic consumption has disastrous consequences for your health. Statistics indicate that heavy drinkers die at least eight years earlier than their moderate drinking friends. Not counted in this loss of eight years are the tremendous emotional and financial losses incurred by alcoholics and their families, and the many additional lost years in terms of poor health. Since we all have such very different tolerances for alcohol, it is up to you to gauge what is "moderate" drinking for your body. It may be less than two drinks per day, and it should not be more. Furthermore, if a whiff of alcohol makes you intoxicated, or if you can't stop drinking once you begin, you are not one of the moderate drinkers who will live longer than an abstainer. You are better off as an abstainer, because drinking in your case does far more harm than good. If you are a heavy drinker, it is urgent that you get yourself into the moderate or abstaining category as soon as possible. Don't kid yourself that your physiological make-up allows you to tolerate three or more drinks a day. You are on the way to becoming an alcoholic, if you are not one already, and the best thing you can do for your own health and your family's peace of mind is to see your doctor or join Alcoholics Anonymous. The alternative is to lose your sanity and your life.

9.
Be Active, Exercise, and Live Longer

A characteristic of most people who have lived to be 90 or 100 is that throughout their lives they have been physically active. Movement and exercise have a direct effect on health. Physical activity conditions the body, helping it to function more efficiently. The heart pumps more blood with each stroke, the lungs move more air with each breath, the arteries develop extra collaterals to reach cells more directly, and the muscles retain more of their mass. Of course, few of the centenarians who have led an active life were aware of the physiological effects of exercise. They simply enjoyed physical activity and experienced a zest for life that resulted from and contributed to their energetic lifestyle.

In a survey of 402 Americans living to be 95 or older, Dr. George Gallup, the originator of the famous Gallup Poll, was impressed by the large number of long-lived individuals who had spent most of their lives working hard at physical labor. He described these select individuals by saying, "They were a highly energized group, men and women who would jump out of bed in the morning feeling not only that the world was their apple but also that they could pare and core it."[1] Perhaps exercise or physical activity caused this zest, but Gallup was not sure which came first, the zest or the exercise. Only 6 percent of this group with an average age of 99 years said that they had ever tired easily. They claimed that they had a lot of stamina, and their activities throughout their lives proved it.

While only a third of Gallup's 402 near-centenarians made an effort to exercise in addition to their work, they were all highly exercised through their occupations. The typical man in this group worked until he was 80 years old, fifteen years past today's routine retirement age. Most of the men worked on their feet at hard physical labor. Almost a third were farmers, and 39 percent worked outdoors as manual laborers. They averaged a work week of almost sixty hours, with a third of them working longer than seventy hours a week. none worked less than forty hours a week. A quarter of the women worked outside their homes, and the rest worked as housewives at a time when labor-saving devices were unknown.

The kind of activity which many of these long-living people experienced throughout their lives is hardly available to contemporary Americans. The old people interviewed by Gallup and his associates were born in the mid-nineteenth century, at a time when most Americans were engaged in far more strenuous kinds of activities than they are today. Although life expectancy at the time when these people were born was only 49 years (primarily due to the absence of modern medicine), Gallup felt that some aspects of their lifestyle were more conducive to long life than the patterns we experience today. The primary difference is in physical activity. Dr. Gallup speculated that due to contemporary Americans' reliance on modern conveniences, there may be fewer centenarians in the next decades. He described with obvious disgust the preoccupation of Americans with labor-saving gadgets in the home and with automobiles, and complained that the world of his centenarians was not the "presto" world of today which seems determined to abolish physical activity—and with it perhaps human beings themselves. "Perhaps we have seen the end to the centenarians in this country," Gallup stated, "perhaps we are at the peak of a cycle that can repeat itself only if Americans strike an intellectual decline that will make the muscle popular—or at least necessary—again."

This doomsday prediction of Dr. George Gallup on the

state of physical activity (or inactivity) in American life was made before President Kennedy launched his physical fitness program and before physical fitness became institutionalized in elementary and secondary schools throughout the United States. The target generations of that program are now adults, who appear to have taken seriously the lessons taught to them in earlier decades. Rather than requiring an intellectual decline to lead to the repopularization of physical activity, it appears that an intellectual awareness of the need for activity is what has motivated people in great numbers to begin jogging, bicycling, swimming, playing tennis, and engaging in a host of other physical activities. That educaton plays a role in longevity is suggested by the fact that few bluecollar workers (who typically have no education beyond high school) participate in aerobic sports, while enthusiasts among the whitecollar group are increasing dramatically in numbers.

According to a recent article in *Newsweek* (May 23, 1977), 87.5 million Americans over the age of 18 claim to participate in athletic activity. This is nearly two-thirds of the adult population of the United States, and articles in both *Newsweek* and *Time* magazines insist that the nation is in the thrall of an unprecedented obsession with physical fitness. No age group appears exempt from what has been called the "great shape-up". Children as young as 3 months are being exposed to "kiddie fit", while corporate executives, housewives, and senior citizens are in increasing numbers participating in formal exercise classes and programs, as well as in informal outdoors activity. It has been estimated that there are 7 to 10 million joggers in the United States and 29 million tennis buffs. Racquetball, a combination of handball and squash, may be replacing tennis as the fastest growing participation sport. The ranks of racquetball enthusiasts have swelled from 50,000 in 1970 to over 3 million in 1977.

The cause of the craze in physical fitness has not been identified. Some have suggested that constant exposure to medical reports of the danger of inactivity to the heart have led people in great numbers to move from being sports spectators to being participants. Others suggest that people are becoming more active just because it feels good. Regardless of the cause, the result may well be the reduction of premature deaths and the extension of life expectancy.

In addition to Gallup's evidence that a great majority of

the long-lived people he interviewed had led active lives, studies comparing members of active and sedentary occupations suggest the importance of activity in longevity. Distinctly higher mortality rates due to heart disease in sedentary workers than in physical workers have been documented in a number of different countries. For example, champion cross-country skiers in Finland lived seven years longer than did the rest of the population. In a recently reported California survey of more than 6,000 longshoremen it was found that those who spent their entire careers doing heavy labor on the docks had half as many heart attacks as did workers who switched to light work or who held sedentary office jobs. Bus drivers in London died younger and had more cardiovascular disease than the more active conductors. British postmen also had fewer heart attacks than their counterparts in Civil Service office jobs.

The active and inactive groups described above may have been unequal in economic status and life habits. In a study designed to control for these differences, the incidence of heart disease was studied during a 15-year period in more than 10,000 men and women in Israeli collective settlements. Regardless of the type of work done in the Kibbutz, socio-economic status is equal. Also, food is prepared for the whole community in one kitchen and served in a communal dining room. Leisure activities are also similar for all members of the group. Thus, activity on the job was one of the few characteristics which differentiated the individuals studied. In all age brackets and in both sexes the sedentary workers had an incidence rate of heart disease about 2 to 3.5 times as high as non-sedentary workers. The argument that people with a predisposition to heart disease might self-select themselves into sedentary work could be raised, but it is difficult to accept that this factor in itself would account for the great differences observed in all age brackets and in both sexes.

However, because there is an element of self-selection involved even in the Israeli study, it is impossible to determine whether activity actually *causes* longer life. People who are healthier and predisposed to live longer in the first place may choose more active jobs. The dock workers and skiers, for example, may be able to stick to their strenuous activity simply because they have been endowed with better cardiovascular systems and general health than the average person.

The research on the association between sleep and longevity is another source suggesting that inactivity leads to shorter life, but this research, like the research on occupational activity is not conclusive. People who are predisposed to live longer may be the ones who feel better and who do not spend a lot of time sleeping. The relationship between sleep and longevity has been demonstrated by Dr. E. Cuyler Hammond working at the American Cancer Society in New York. Dr. Hammond was director of a project which involved collecting information on health patterns, lifestyle, and mortality of over a million people in the United States to obtain clues about the causes of cancer and to identify people at high risk for any chronic diseases. Almost seventy thousand Cancer Society volunteers collected information in 1959 and helped to follow up on subjects each year for the next six years. Results in the first years of the project were similar to results over the six-year period in identifying a relationship between longer life and sleeping six to eight hours per day. People who said that they slept nine hours or more had higher mortality rates, and the mortality rates for people sleeping more than ten hours were very high. It is possible that part of the reason that mortality was so high was that excessive sleeping involved too much inactivity. Forcing young, healthy people to stay in bed resting constantly for a two-week period leads to physiological changes in the heart, lungs, and muscles which imitate the changes occurring in old age. Such observations have led Dr. Herbert deVires, an exercise physiologist at the University of Southern California, to suggest that many of the deleterious physiological changes in old age may result as much from disuse as from biological aging.

Too little sleep was also shown to have negative consequences in the study directed by Dr. Hammond. Sleeping less than six hours a night was associated with slightly increased mortality, and getting less than four or five hours had a greatly increased risk of death. Does this mean that too much activity is unhealthful? Such a conclusion is doubtful. It is more likely that the people reporting less than four or five hours sleep a night were experiencing serious problems preventing them from sleeping, or they were otherwise stressing their bodies to the point where they could not compensate.

This research suggests that moderate sleeping habits are best. Data collected in this manner also highlight the difficulty of determining the *causes* of long life. The data suggest that inactivity may be related to an earlier death, but they do not provide us with certainly about that conclusion.

While there are no studies on humans which prove undeniably that physical activity leads to longer life, the evidence points strongly in that direction. Physically inactive people die younger to such a reliable degree that physical activity can be used as a strong predictor of longevity. People who are active live longer, and there are clear benefits to health which could serve to prevent cardiovascular disease as a result of exercise. A study of physical fitness among male employees of the Metropolitan Life Insurance Company indicated the value of regular exercise. Employees who engaged in sports and physical activities providing challenge to the cardiovascular system did well on the physical fitness test, while those who were heavy smokers, overweight, and physically inactive did poorly. Upon completion of the test, a physical fitness counselor informed each employee of the category (above average, average, or below average) in which his performance had placed him. For those who did poorly on the test, recommendations were made by the counselor to assist the employee in developing a practical reconditioning program that fitted in with his lifestyle. Indeed, the Metropolitan Life Insurance Company and a number of other large firms are already acting on the evidence which suggests that activity improves health and longevity. Businesses are subsidizing exercise programs for employees in an effort to improve health. Such efforts are not completely altruistic. Employees who exercise instead of drinking at lunch are more productive in the afternoon, and they are far less likely to require payouts from company-financed health insurance. Thus, the evidence that physical fitness improves longevity is conclusive enough to convince big business to invest in exercise programs for employees.

The physiological benefits of exercise are well-documented. Exercise increases the strength of the heart muscle and its ability to pump blood throughout the body. It stimulates the development of collateral circulation when the coronary blood flow is impaired by atherosclerosis, and it can reduce heart rate and blood pressure. Increase in the proportion of body muscle to body fat is achieved through exercise, and this effect coupled with the likelihood of weight loss through exercise works to lower the levels of fat in the blood, the blood pressure, and the work load on the heart. Regular exercising may also serve to cause people to give up smoking and to reduce their eating and drinking. You can't have two martinis and a big lunch if you jog at noon.

Exercise also reduces tension. Dr. Herbert deVries and his associates at the University of Southern California have demonstrated that exercise as moderate as a brisk fifteen minute walk has the same effect as a tranquilizer on muscular tension. Thus, while studies comparing active and inactive workers do not definitively demonstrate that activity causes longer life, there are physiological effects resulting from exercise which lead us to believe that the relationship is a causal one. Studies of members of long-lived societies and of animals also suggest a causal relationship between activity and longevity.

An effort has been made to study the lifestyles of longevous peoples for the "secret" to their long life. In parts of the world such as Abkhasia in the U.S.S.R., where whole groups of people have extraordinarily long life expectancies, activity has been documented to be one of the secrets which differentiates these people. Since everyone there is physically active from an early age and since most of the people live longer than the rest of the Russian population, the problem that only the healthiest choose active occupations is avoided. Physical activity coupled with their moderate eating habits seems to be extending the Abkhasians' life expectancy.

In her book describing life in Abkhasia, Professor Sula Benet of Hunter College points out that retirement is a status unknown in Abkhasian thinking. From the beginning of life until its end, an Abkhasian does what he or she is capable of doing, and this involves physical labor. They consider physical work to be vital to life. Physical endurance is not stretched beyond capacity, but the body is pushed to be as active as possible without stress.

Dr. Benet quotes what Abkhasians say, "Without rest, a man cannot work; without work, the rest does not give you any benefit."[3]

Dr. Benet feels that the Abkhasian attitude toward physical activity may be as important as the activity itself. When they are children, they do what they are capable of doing, progressing from the easiest to the most strenuous tasks. When they age the curve reverses, but they never stop working completely. They do what they can at their own pace. At no point in the life span does an Abkhasian become sedentary. They feel that inactivity is bad for well-being, and that it is better to move without purpose than to sit still. Such attitudes keep them healthy.

However, the scientific purist, looking for the perfect study to demonstrate a causal relationship between activity and longevity would not be satisfied with the evidence provided by the Abkhasians. While everyone is active and lives longer, there are other factors such as diet, lack of stress in life, and good genetic background which probably contribute to the Abkhasians' long life. Thus, the role of physical activity in extending life expectancy in this group is not clear cut. The magnitude of the effect cannot be measured. There are no human studies which can satisfy such a purist because humans cannot be equated genetically (except in the case of identical twins), and because humans cannot be randomly assigned to conditions of activity and inactivity. Only animal studies can meet these stringent criteria, and it is with animal studies that we have the most convincing evidence that physical activity extends life expectancy. In both rats and mice, it has been shown that exercise increases life expectancy. This finding has been replicated in a number of laboratories and is accepted now as an established fact. Given the suggestive evidence in humans and the conclusive evidence in rats that longevity is extended through exercise, what are the kinds of exercise which should be undertaken to prolong life, and at what age must such a regimen begin?

PRESCRIPTION OF EXERCISE FOR HEALTH AND LONGEVITY

Ideally, we should follow the example of the Abkhasians who begin by stressing the importance of activity early in life and never stop valuing its importance. In this light the growing number of programs in the United States encouraging fitness in pre-school age children is an encouraging sign. On the other hand, it's never too late to receive positive health benefits from physical exercise. Until a few years ago this fact was not understood, and the converse was believed. Exercise physiologists argued that unless activity had been undertaken in young adulthood or before, and maintained throughout life, the benefits of exercise were nil. Indeed, it was thought that exercise in old age was harmful. Over the last two decades, Dr. Herbert deVries working with older men and women in Laguna Hills, California, has demonstrated that exercise can have beneficial physiological effects when undertaken at any age—even in the late eighties. This does not mean that we should all rush immediately into a program of strenuous exercise. Dr. deVries and a number of exercise physiologists believe that exercise should be individually prescribed as scrupulously as drugs are prescribed.

Dr. deVries has set a number of steps through which the prospective exerciser must proceed. The first step in the prescription of exercise is a visit to the doctor's office. After the patient's history has been taken and a thorough physical examination performed, the patient should be assessed in an exercise stress test including the recording of heart activity (electrocardiogram or EKG) during exercise. Such a test involves pedaling a stationary bike or walking vigorously on a treadmill while being monitored until symptoms like breathlessness or chest pains occur. This test measures the body's capacity for work and detects otherwise silent heart disease. Such a test can be compared to running a car motor to find the problem. Looking at the car while it is idle, like examining a patient at rest, can lead the mechanic to miss important problems with the engine. It is only when the machine is tested while operating that many significant difficulties can be detected.

Not all physicians have the facilities to give stress tests in their offices, but they will be able to refer you to a clinic or an exercise physiologist who can perform this service. The fee is usually under $50 and sometimes less than $30. Many believe that because so many Americans have undetected cardiovascular disease, everyone over the age of 45 should have a stress test whether they plan to exercise or not. For potential exercise enthusiasts who cannot be bothered with seeing a doctor before hurling themselves into exercise—these individuals are being very unwise—some physicians have advised the "talk test." If you cannot hold a conversation while performing the exercise because you are out of breath, then you are overdoing it.

In addition to helping you determine if it is safe for you to exercise, a stress test provides you with information about how hard you should push your body. Stress tests push individuals to approach their maximum capacity, and using this estimate of maximum capacity, a person learns what heart rate should not be exceeded while performing exercise. After a warm-up period of five to ten minutes, strenuous exercise can be undertaken in such a way that the individual does not exceed 70 to 85 percent of maximum capacity. This maximum rate can be estimated by a person's age, but it is much safer to have it estimated by the actual stress test. The age method involves starting with a rate of 220 beats per minute and subtracting your age. Thus, if you are 40, this estimate of your maximum capacity is 180 beats per minute. Seventy to 85 percent of that capacity is 126 to 153 beats per minute, the heart rate which should not be exceeded during strenuous exercise for a 40-year-old. Individuals should learn to take their pulse rate and check it with a second hand periodically during the exercise period.

After the physical examination and stress test, the doctor is ready to prescribe the exercise. Benefits to the cardiovascular system come largely from aerobic, isotonic, or dynamic forms of exercise. Such exercise as running, jogging, brisk walking, bicycling, dancing, skating, and cross-country skiing—which involve the big muscles of the body and relatively long, continuous performance—are the kinds of exercise that get the heart pumping, expand the blood vessels, and increase the flow of oxygen-bearing blood. Many physicians and exercise physiologists feel that swimming is the most perfect form of aerobic exercise because it does not jar the body or produce muscle and joint injuries. Benefits are less from sprinting because it does not last long enough to get the heart pumping blood throughout the body, and from tennis, especially doubles, because activity is not continuous enough unless the players are really proficient at the game.

Weekend exercising is not sufficient for conditioning and may, in fact, lead to injury and undue stress to the body. Unless you exercise at least three times spread over a week, for at least half an hour each time, forget it. You will do more harm than good.

After exercise has been prescribed and the patient has used his exercise prescription for six weeks during which time he keeps a daily record of his heart rate response to the prescription, a second visit to the doctor's office is in order. At this time a retest on the stress test is carried out. If regression or no improvement has occurred in the patient's maximum capacity, a physical examination should be performed to rule out disease. If suitable improvement is shown, the exercise prescription should be adjusted upward accordingly. In any case, at this six-week check-up, a new prescription should be made, and the patient is then allowed to work on the new prescription for the next twelve weeks. The third and final visit in this series to the doctor's office occurs after this twelve-week period. If the patient has shown improvement on the third exercise stress test, he or she can be released with final written instructions for future adjustments to the exercise regimen and advised to return in a year for the annual physical examination. If there is no improvement or if there is regression, a physical examination should again be undertaken to rule out disease, and the prescription should be modified downward if no disease is found. The unimproved patient needs a fourth visit six weeks later before discharge for a year of exercise until the next office visit.

Dr. deVries' prescription of exercise was devised for people who have not engaged in strenuous exercise for some years, who are presumably out of shape, and who are older. It is admittedly a conservative approach to exercising, but it is safe. Younger people who believe that they can undertake an exercise regimen without so much consultation with the physician should at least have an initial check-up or not be too many months past their annual physical exam before dramatically increasing their activity. Remember that even trained athletes occasionally die from over-exertion, and youth is not exempt. Training should be gradual so that you do not over-tax your system and so that your muscles and joints do not become so painful as a result of exercise that you quit altogether. For a good and well-tested program, you might want to select the Royal Canadian Air Force Exercise Program (available in paperback), or one of the aerobics programs of Dr. Kenneth Cooper (described in his books, *Aerobics* and *Aerobics for Women*, the latter co-authored with Mildred Cooper). All of these programs involve graduated stages of exercise designed to condition an individual at a safe pace.

For older individuals (it has been found that exercise is both safe and beneficial for men and women over the age of 55), Dr. deVries has developed the following program of exercise based on their capacity to improve the cardiovascular and pulmonary systems. The program has three parts: static-stretching exercises, calisthenic exercises, and a modified jogging program. This program was devised to be both safe and effective in improving physical work capacity. Calisthenic exercises which might contribute to muscular strength, muscular endurance, and flexibility have been selected. For improvement of the heart and lung systems, a jogging (run-walk) regimen was devised which has a low intensity entry point and a very gradual progression suitable for unconditioned people over 60. To prevent muscular soreness to the greatest extent possible, and also to improve joint mobility, static-stretching techniques are used which have been proved to be effective for these purposes.

The first exercises to be carried out in this program are the static-stretching exercises pictured in Figure 6. Each position should be held for a one-minute period, and in exercises 2, 4, and 5, intermediate positions can be used until such time as improved flexibility allows the use of the final position illustrated. After each exercise, you should rest until your heart rate recovers to within 10 beats per minute of its resting value. Rest five minutes before undertaking the calisthenics. The second step of the program involves the calisthenics picture in Figure 7. They should each be done for around two minutes at the following cadences: (1) toe touchers, 3 repetitions per minute; (2) modified sit-ups, 7 per minute; (3) alternate leg raisers, 8 per minute, and (4) modified push-ups, 4 per minute. Again, heart rate should be allowed to return to within 10 beats per minute of its resting value after each exercise. After a ten-minute rest period, the jogging part of the program can begin. Establish your own natural walking and running rates, and carry out five sets of running 50 steps, then walking 50 steps. Heart rate should be measured by feeling your pulse for the last thirty seconds of each run phase. Then, before undertaking the next run-walk sequence, let your heart rate drop to within 10 beats per minute of its resting value.

FIGURE 6. Static-stretching Exercises.

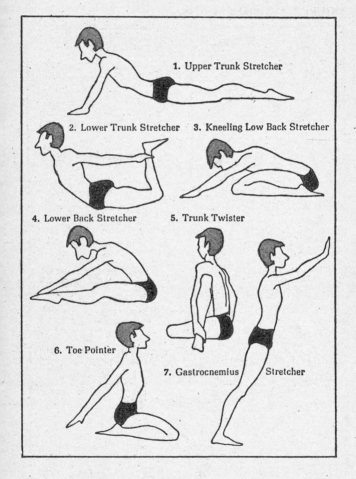

1. Upper Trunk Stretcher
2. Lower Trunk Stretcher
3. Kneeling Low Back Stretcher
4. Lower Back Stretcher
5. Trunk Twister
6. Toe Pointer
7. Gastrocnemius Stretcher

SOURCE: H. A. deVries, "Prescription of Exercises for Older Men from Telemetered Exercise Heart Rate Data," *Geriatrics*, 1971, 26, 102–111. © 1971 by Harcourt Brace, Jovanovich, Inc.

FIGURE 7. Calisthenics Exercises.

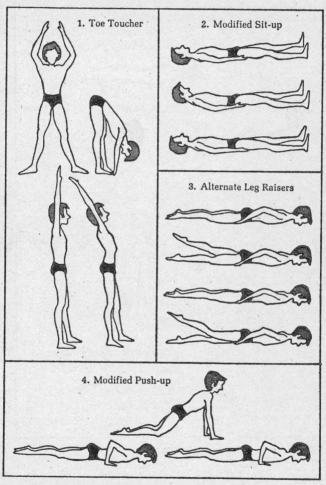

For cadence used, see text discussion.
SOURCE: H. A. deVries, "Prescription of Exercise for Older Men from Tele-metered Exercise Heart Rate Data," *Geriatrics*, 1971, 25, 102–111. © 1971 by Harcourt Brace, Jovanovich, Inc.

Dr. deVries feels that for normal people above the age of 60, the maximum heart rate should be set at 145 beats per minute. Sizable improvements in oxygen pulse, ventilation, and vital capacity were seen in his experimental subjects for whom this was set as maximum, and it is also possible that the maximum heart rate could be set lower without compromising the rate of improvement. Indeed, in other research, deVries found that for all but the most highly conditioned people over the age of 60, vigorous walking which raises heart rate to 100 to 120 beats per minute for thirty to sixty minutes daily constitutes a sufficient stimulus to bring about some, although possibly not optimal, improvement in the heart and lung systems.

Exercise provides many benefits for young and old alike. In addition to the probable effect on longevity, exercise has clear psychological benefits as well. The participants in Dr. deVries studies report an increase in general vigor and energy level. They feel better—more like jumping out of bed in the morning. Some reported that their sex lives improved as a result of their increased physical exercise. While Dr. deVries is quick to point out that he did not empirically document any such effect, he is not alone in hearing people who have become engaged in a regular exercise program report that their desire and capacity for sexual activity has increased. One reason for this may be that they are more relaxed. Exercise has a tranquilizing effect equal to the effect of a Miltown. In a relatively unconditioned individual, as little as a fifteen-minute walk which raises heart rate to only 100 beats per minute can have relaxing effects lasting for at least an hour. Greater tension reduction is undoubtedly received with more exercise. Marathon runners who push themselves beyond three miles describe with surprising consistency a feeling of euphoria as they continue running. They report experiencing a "high" which they describe as a very pleasant state which motivates them to push through the pain of early fatigue to reach this twilight state. Additionally it has been found that chronically depressed people show a gradual reduction in their symptoms when they get involved in an exercise regimen.

Thus, for health and for psychological well-being—not to mention the positive cosmetic features of physical activity—take up some form of exercise and live longer. You will live better as well.

EDUCATION
AND OCCUPATION

10.
Does Education
Extend Your Life?

இ◦There is ample evidence demonstrating that people with more education live longer. The death rate for people with less than eight years of schooling is considerably higher than the death rate for the population in general, while the death rate for graduates of college is impressively less than the rate for the general population. There is at least a five-year difference in life expectancy between college graduates and eighth grade drop-outs.

A brief look at such data might lead us to believe that education extends life expectancy, but the answer is just not that simple. Education is confounded with other socioeconomic variables which in themselves are related to longer life. For example, people in the middle and upper classes live considerably longer than people in the lower class. This results from differences in opportunity between rich and middle-income people versus poor people. It is also possible that the gene pool for longevity is more favorable in the higher social status groups. To answer the question of whether you should return to school to extend your life, let us examine more closely the statistics on education and longevity.

Longevity is dramatically influenced by a set of highly related factors which determine an individual's social class.

147

The three major components of social class are occupation, income, and education. They are interrelated in a very complex manner which tends to perpetuate differences in social class. From birth, children of parents in higher social classes have more advantages, including the opportunity to attend better schools. Their parents, who have most likely had more than the average level of education, feel positively about education and encourage the children to do well in school. Good performance in the elementary school years places the children in the "college prep" classes in high school which in turn fulfills college entrance requirements. Once into college, avenues to higher status jobs open. Indeed, college education is required for almost all of the higher status jobs in our society. Higher status jobs bring higher incomes and make it possible for individuals to purchase numerous resources advantageous to longer life.

Higher status and higher salaried positions are better for your health. Such positions carry fewer on-the-job risks—that is, individuals are less frequently exposed to hazards and situations in which dangerous accidents can occur. Fatigue, inorganic dusts (in substances such as silica and asbestos), absorption of poisons, excessive heat, and sudden variations in temperature and dampness are less common in whitecollar jobs than blue collar ones. As a result, the risk of serious or fatal accidents is lower and general health is better for professional level workers. Health benefits are often better for whitecollar workers as well. Higher status positions also have more liberal sick-leave benefits so that it is not necessary to remain on the job when the individual is sick and should be nursing his or her health.

In addition to placing people in healthier jobs, higher education makes them more likely to be aware of proper health care and nutrition. As a result of this sensitization to health factors, they may take better care of themselves. Resources such as food, clothing, housing, and medical care are also more easily afforded by people of higher social status. Poor people who have had little education and who are not quali- tors involved in the relationship between education and longevity. More physically and mentally competent people are fied to undertake better paying, highly skilled jobs have little access to resources conducive to longevity, thus they die younger. In societies in which there is less social class distinction and less poverty than is found in the United States (such as in the Scandinavian countries), life expectancy is longer.

Environmental factors related to greater longevity in people of higher social class are not, however, the only factors involved in the relationship between education and longevity. More physically and mentally competent people are more likely to complete college and graduate studies, and are usually selected to occupy higher status occupations. This result may well be due to a genetic effect that combines with the effect of social class. The genetically superior with respect to longevity are better able to elbow their way into the more protected and lucrative occupational roles, which in turn augment even further any genetic predisposition to longevity. This genetic factor (discussed in Chapter 4) not only favors longevity in its own right, but also indirectly favors longer life by inducing a more favorable environment such as is associated with higher occupational status.

We will discuss occupation and its effect on longevity in Chapter 11, with the caution that it is really impossible to separate the effects of education, occupation, and income.

While the life expectancy test in Chapter 1 associates about the same number of years of life expectancy with occupation and with education, the effects of the two factors simply cannot be considered as totally independent. For example, professional workers who live from three to five years longer than the general population are the same people who are studied in research on education and longevity and found to live five or more years longer. It would not be appropriate to add ten years to the life expectancies of these people (which would be the result if the statistics on education and occupation were treated as completely separate effects). However, attributing some years of life expectancy to both occupation and education is reasonable, since people of somewhat different educational background often perform the same job. Furthermore, income is not always equal for the same job and the same level of education. Dr. Evelyn M. Kitagawa and Dr. Philip M. Hauser reviewed the key finding of three major research undertakings of the Population Research Center in which they were involved at the University of Chicago. They were able to demonstrate that education, occupation, and income all had independent effects on longevity, and that is why we have made each of the three categories into separate questions on the longevity test. Drs. Kitagawa and Hauser believe that of the three factors, education is the most significant.

THE SIGNIFICANCE OF EDUCATION IN LONGEVITY

Scholars have been aware of the relationship between education and longevity for many years. A study reported by the Metropolitan Life Insurance Company on college graduates in 1932 demonstrated that at the time of graduation the life expectancy of the college graduates was five years longer than the population as a whole. This study is still one of the most definitive on education and life expectancy. The study traced the subsequent life history of nearly 40,000 men (including more than 6,000 who graduated with honors and almost 5,000 athletes) after they graduated from eight Eastern colleges in the classes of 1870 to 1905. The data in that study involved college graduates over 100 years ago. These people were an especially select group in that less than 5 percent of the population attended college in the 19th and early 20th centuries. Today, fully half of the population get at least some college experience, a much less select group. However, recent data still indicate that college graduates live longer.

Metropolitan Life Insurance Company statistics published in 1975 indicate that people who attended college between 1900 and 1960 live considerably longer than the national average. In another study 270,000 men employed by the Bell System Operating Companies were surveyed in the late 1960's. Those who entered the organization with a college degree had a lower heart attack rate, disability rate, and death rate than those with less education. This effect occurred at every age, in every part of the United States, and in all of the various departments of the organization. Thus, if we take these data and add them to the information gathered in the Metropolitan Life Insurance Company studies, it appears that education level has been related to longevity for at least 100 years. Athletes among the college graduates had only a slightly greater advantage over the nonathlete college graduates, but the honor men had a two-year advantage over the rest of the college graduates at the age of 22. Hence, men graduating with honors from college, presumably the brightest and most likely men to succeed, could expect when they graduated to live seven years longer than the average 22-year-old American male in 1900.

Thus, people of greater intelligence attend college, and the brightest among these intelligent people—the honors graduates—lives longest. As noted earlier, a number of studies have produced results which suggest a genetic component in the relationship between intelligence and longevity. This genetic factor probably accounts for some of the relationship between education and longevity. Since very bright individuals are likely to be of a genetic make-up which predisposes them to be healthier and live longer, it is the genetic effect rather than the education effect which is leading to longer life. Additionally, bright people are more likely to be able to handle life realistically and constructively. They learn best how to take advantage of all that is known and available to them to maintain health, growth, and favorable life circumstances. In the sense that education is an index of high intelligence, it is not causing longer life. It is merely associated with a factor leading to longer life.

As far as returning to school and increasing your level of education—that may or may not affect the number of years you live. Of course, the younger you are, the more years of your life will be influenced by greater education and its advantages. In this sense, the younger you are, the more likely it is that returning to school will extend the length of your life. Quantity of life is not all that is influenced by education, however. At any age, returning to school will enhance the quality of life—adding life to years, even if it does not add years to life. For this reason we should all be involved with educational activities throughout our lives.

EDUCATION AND THE QUALITY OF LIFE

Over twenty years ago it was asserted that as a consequence of the lengthening of life expectancy and the acceleration of change in society, this country needed educational programming throughout life. In 1971 the Carnegie Commission on Higher Education gave emphasis to this point by stating:

Society would gain if work and study were mixed throughout a life-time, thus reducing the sense of sharply compartment-

alized roles of isolated students. The sense of isolation would
be reduced if more students were also workers and if more
workers could also be students; if the aged mixed on the
job and in the classroom in a more normally structured
type of community; if all members of the community value
both study and work and had a better chance to understand
the flow of life from youth to age. Society would be more
integrated across the lines that now separate students and
workers, youth and age.[1]

Education throughout life enhances human development and
provides means to develop the individual's abilities,
knowledge, skills, and character.

Many individuals are skeptical of formal education and are
delighted to leave school and never to return. Such attitudes
reflect inadequacies in our educational system, such as an emphasis on grades instead of learning. Educational institutions
have also come under criticism because it has been felt that
what goes on in schools is not relevant to the problems and
issues of society and of daily life. One of the ways for educational institutions to become a more integral and relevant
part of society is to take a life span approach—opening the
doors to people in middle and late adulthood as well as to
youth. The present inoculation model of education, in which
an individual receives a sufficient dose of education early in
life thereby immunizing him or her from the need for additional formal learning, is obsolete. Change is too rapid in the
20th century for concepts learned twenty years previously to
remain intact.

There are a number of reasons for educational institutions
to attend more to the needs of adults of all ages, and there is
also evidence that educators are doing just that. For one
thing, as a result of the dropping birth rate in the United
States, fewer children are entering school. We expanded our
educational facilities dramatically to meet the needs of the
very large generation of individuals born after World War II.
Now that those children have reached maturity, we have an
overabundance of classroom space and trained teachers who
can devote themselves to teaching adults. While there are
fewer youth available to be taught, there are a growing number of adults in society who want and need additional education.

Since many middle-aged people are deciding to change

careers and many women are deciding to begin careers after they raise their children, a large group of middle-aged people are returning to school for degrees. This phenomenon of more adults in educational institutions is a result of the greater number of years people are surviving in the 1970's, and the fulfillment and interest education provides for these individuals may cause them to live even longer—and better.

Expanding educational philosophy to cover the life span can improve the quality of life in terms of alleviating deprivation in those who have not had educational advantages, in terms of enriching the lives of people of all ages and educational levels, and in terms of preventing future generations from suffering from lack of education.

The alleviation of educational deprivation can occur at any point in adulthood, and many programs are available to provide people with entry into higher level jobs by allowing them to complete high school or college degrees. Such programs can also lessen the differences between generations in terms of the level of education attained. Like the poor and the members of ethnic and other minority groups, the aged in our country suffer from educational deprivation. Educational deprivation in the aged is absolute inasmuch as almost two-thirds of the people over 65 have no more than an eighth grade education. Deprivation is relative as well, because old people were educated in the early 1900's when a very different knowledge base existed. While many people think that intelligence declines with age because of their own experience with older people, psychologists have demonstrated that intelligence remains stable over most of the life span. The reason many older people seem less sharp is because they have had much less education, and they went to school fifty or more years ago. Education for large proportions of the older population might affect our image of the aged and make us recognize more clearly the value of their thinking and experience. This in turn would increase our expectations of our own capacities in later life making us optimistic rather than depressed about our own aging.

The elderly do respond to educational opportunities. For example, the Institute of Lifetime Learning sponsored by the American Association of Retired Persons (AARP) and the National Retired Teachers Association (NRTA) reports a wide range of courses for older adults and impressive enrollments that would not generally be included in national educational statistics. Since its inception in 1964, the Institute has offered courses on more than 100 topics in over a dozen locations across the country. Thousands of elderly students have enrolled in these courses and in correspondence courses, and additional hundreds of thousands have been reached through courses broadcast over the radio. As we will see in later chapters, having a purpose in life and having interesting activities in which to participate appears to increase the number of years we live. Learning to paint or to write poetry at the age of 70 or 80 is the kind of opportunity enjoyed by participants in the Institute of Lifetime Learning—and such opportunities clearly enhance life.

The Institute of Lifetime Learning is a privately financed educational center. Today, however, it is not just private educational institutions which are opening their doors to older people. Serious consideration is being given in some states to the prospect of extensive programs of education for the aged. The president of the University of Hawaii in an address to the state legislature stated that a senior citizen's bill of educational rights should be passed. His basic thought was that an individual who has completed his or her period of employed work life, and thereby made a contribution to society through products and taxes, should be entitled to an earned period of time in educational institutions to further his or her development. This is a philosophy similar to that of the post World War II GI Bill of Rights in which the returning soldier was entitled, after his service, to a period of free education in a program of his choice. Why not, by analogy, several years of free education to individuals who have completed their service to society through their work life and careers?

Some states have adopted the essence of this proposal by providing free tuition in community colleges to students over the age of 65. Many colleges and universities have large continuing education programs. Remarkable among them are the programs of the New School for Social Research in New York City and the Continuing Education Program at the University of California at Los Angeles. Hundreds of thousands of adults have extended their education through these two programs alone, and these programs on the East and West Coasts are serving as models for universities and colleges throughout the country. Undergraduate and graduate degree programs are also much more open to students over the age of thirty than they have been in the past. And why not? The average thirty-year-old has forty-five years left to live—over half of his or her life.

Prevention of inequities resulting from differences in educational opportunity is one way that educational intervention could affect life expectancy as well as the quality of life. By providing more equal opportunities for individuals of all social statuses to attain a college degree, and hence to enter into higher occupational categories, life expectancy would increase as it has in Scandinavian countries. Educational intervention in later life may also add years by preventing difficulties of adjustment in middle and old age. For example, retiring individuals who derived their identity from their occupation face a difficult adjustment when their self image as a productive member of society is lost. Such life crises are at least partially implicated in the high incidence of suicide in older white males. Courses in pre-retirement planning stress the development of interests and hobbies outside the job to carry people over the stress of retirement. Interests which can bcome full-time pursuits in the absence of employment can be developed through education. Attending classes in itself is an activity providing interaction with others and meaning and stimulation in the lives of people who are retired. Of course, one need not wait until retirement to seek this stimulation—it should be a life-long pattern.

Another way in which education might positively affect longevity would be in introducing elementary school children to concepts and information about the human cycle. In the Abkhasian society, long life is an accepted fact, and children are familiar with old people and taught to give the highest respect to those who have lived the longest. Furthermore, children learn to expect to live a long life themselves, and much of their youth is spent in eager anticipation of the joys and status of being older. Such training is in no way a part of young Americans' experience, either in the home or in the school. Because of this the young are not provided with a perspective on the life span which would be more appropriate to the changing culture in which they live. There are more old people in contemporary society than ever before, and the youth of today will themselves survive to a very advanced age. They could learn to anticipate this later period of their lives with pleasure rather than with disgust and fear. Education is a means to provide them with such a perspective, and if we would use it in this manner, it would have an even greater impact than it currently has on the quality of life.

The answer to the question posed in this chapter—"Does education extend your life?"—is complicated. Simply stated, we do not know for sure. People with more education live longer, and this is partly a result of the fact that they attain higher occupational status and greater income. Thus, if you are relatively young and want to upgrade your occupation, returning to school is likely to extend your life through the advantages you will gain from an advanced degree. In middle and later life, it is less likely that education will have this effect, but continued involvement in educational activities will affect the quality of the remaining years. Since active, stimulated people are the ones who live the longest, life expectancy may even be affected indirectly in this manner. By making yourself a more interesting and interested person, you will create new friendships, activities, and roles. You will be happier and less prone to depression and stress—characteristics which tend to shorten life.

In the end, it is quality rather than quantity of live which interests us most—and education undoubtedly enhances life's quality. From this perspective, the question, "Does education extend your life?" must be answered with an unqualified YES!

11.
Work, Retirement, and Life Expectancy

In the previous chapter it became apparent that social class, which is determined by education, occupation, and income, has a great deal to do with how long we live. By choosing a certain course very early in life, often when we are in high school, we determine to some extent our life expectancy. The work we do, the conditions under which the work is done, and the income derived from that work set certain limits on the style of life we lead. Place and type of residence, quality and abundance of clothes, nutrition of diet, quality of health care, and amount and type of recreational activities are all determined by our job and income.

There appears to be almost a perfect relationship between social class and longevity. The higher the social status, the longer the life. Almost without exception, people working at the highest professional levels (called "Class I" by demographers), such as scientists, lawyers, architects, and physicians, live longer than people in other occupational groups. Farmers are one non-professional group with exceedingly long life expectancy. The clergy—particularly Protestant ministers—also seem to enjoy longer than average lives. At the opposite end of the continuum are those who work in the mines and factories and at other dangerous, heavy labor jobs (identified as

Class V). Those individuals can expect to live a shorter time than average, and their mortality rate is two to three times that of whitecollar workers. Between these two extremes are spread intermediate occupations such as technical, administrative, and managerial workers (Class II); proprietors, clerical, sales, and skilled workers (Class III); and semi-skilled workers (Class IV). These three occupational categories are associated with decreasing—but around average—life expectancy.

The Metropolitan Life Insurance Company currently bases its evaluation of mortality rate by social class on two major studies, one carried out in the United States in 1950 by the Department of Health, Education, and Welfare, and one carried out in England and Wales in 1961 by the Registrar General. A third study, based on employee groups covered by Metropolitan Group Life Insurance between 1965 and 1971, is in agreement with the American and British statistics of previous decades. In all studies, the mortality rates tended to be inversely related to social class. Mortality rates at the lowest level (Class V) were dramatically greater than at higher levels, particularly for the younger age groups (ages 20-24). At the older ages (after 45) the factors affecting longevity appeared to be less related to social class than to biological and genetic influences. Hence, life expectancy after age 45 is not very different between the different socioeconomic groups. This suggests a survival of the fittest model with the selection pressures being much greater in the lower social classes. If a Class V individual survives beyond the age of 45, he or she is at least as well-endowed genetically as an individual in Classes I or II, and will be about as likely to live on into old age as the individual in the higher socioeconomic bracket. Unfortunately, many more of the Class V people are eliminated in the earlier ages which means that their mortality rate is twice to three times as great.

In the United States, race and social class are highly related, and the steep mortality gradient in lower class individuals is reflected in the fact that non-white individuals with the exception of Orientals, have a much shorter life expectancy. Four percent of whites were in Class I according to the HEW study, while only 0.5 percent of none-whites were in this professional category. Conversely, 8 percent of whites were in Class V as opposed to 31 percent of non-whites. The majority of whites were in Classes I, II, and III, while the majority of non-whites were in Classes IV and V. The racial difference in longevity is getting smaller, but it is clear that socioeconomic factors are still highly unfavorable to non-whites. More than any other factor, social class is responsible for the five-year difference in life expectancy between whites and non-whites. While disparities between Class I and Classs II-IV have tended to narrow in recent years, a wide difference still remains between Classes I-IV and Class V.

That the hazards of a given occupation do not account entirely for the higher mortality rate in that socioeconomic level is indicated by the fact that the mortality of wives of various social classes follows the mortality of their husbands. Lifestyle and living environment as well as occupation account for longevity differences between social classes. This is further confirmed by infant mortality rates. The higher the social class, the smaller percentage of infants die in the first year.

In Chapter 2 we discussed the rise in the standard of living, the improvement in public health systems, and the advances in medicine and science which have contributed to increasing life expectancy in the U.S. Further advances may come by providing better access to medical treatment among the socially disadvantaged. At the present time, however, socioeconomic differences in longevity still persist, and it is essential to understand the causes of these differences if we are to provide all Americans with the opportunity of living to be 100.

Relationships between occupation and length of life are not simple. Whether we enjoy long life and good health or whether we become disabled and weak early in our lives and die at an early age depends on many factors which have led us to and which result from our choice of occupation. The environment into which we are born plays a great role, along with our families and the opportunities and heredity with which they provided us. If we attain a position such that our work is comprised of heavy labor, a number of factors cause us to be at risk for a shorter life. For one thing, the chance of accidents on the job is greater than for the average person. In addition, we may be exposed to more pollutants which increases our chances for cancer and other chronic diseases. Our jobs provide a meager income which deprives us and our families of a number of life-prolonging features. Food and clothing are apt to be inadequate. Living conditions may be crowded and unsanitary. If sick leave benefits are minimal, we may continue working while suffering from poor health long after we should quit and seek medical advice and treatment. Furthermore, even if we stop work, we will not have sufficient means to afford the best medical care. Such a picture appears incongruous with earlier discussions of the great strides we have made in extending life expectancy. However, the fact remains that the United States ranks 16th in the world in terms of male life expectancy at birth, and 8th in the world in terms of female life expectancy at birth. This occurs primarily because socioeconomic status is spread very unevenly in our population. Life expectancy in the richest nation in the world is not the best because we have too many poor people.

HAZARDS IN LOWER STATUS OCCUPATIONS

Accidents from dangerous machinery and unsafe processes, the inhalation of harmful dusts of various kinds, the absorption of powerful poisons, the necessity of working in excessively hot, cold, or humid places, and the physical strain of heavy labor are all avoided by individuals working in professional and technical jobs. From the standpoint of physical dangers, there is no question that whitecollar work is safer, and although the psychological stress of whitecollar work takes its toll, the mortality rates still suggest that the physical dangers of bluecollar jobs lead to more deaths than the psychological dangers of whitecollar work.

While a moderate level of physical work throughout life appears to be beneficial for agrarian groups such as the Abkhasians of Russia, very hard labor in mid and late life has been shown to shorten life expectancy. From the age 40 to 45 years and older there appears to be a relation between death rate and amount of energy expended, even when there are no hazards involved. Fatigue caused by very hard work leads to premature death.

Of course, not all industrial jobs are hazardous, as was pointed out by one longevity expert, Dr. Louis Dublin, who insisted that many men gainfully employed in industry are no more exposed to risk than are their mothers and wives at home. Furthermore, working conditions in the 1970's are safer than in previous decades, and measures are continually being legislated to improve occupational safety even more. Nevertheless, the status quo in the United States in which laborers have a mortality rate two to three times greater than the average individual is not acceptable. We must continue to upgrade the living standards and working conditions of lower socioeconomic groups and eliminate the gap in life expectancy between social classes. That this is possible is exemplified in a country such as the Netherlands in which differentials in mortality by social class are hardly apparent. When people enjoy economic advantages, they live longer. This is clear in our own country, and everywhere in the world.

LIFE EXPECTANCY IN PROFESSIONAL AND ELITE GROUPS

It has not been possible to collect information on life expectancy for every occupational group because recent data of this type are not available. The strategy has been rather to compare broad categories of occupation which are related to socioeconomic level to enable you to examine your own chances of survival. To make the point even more clearly that life expectancy varies directly with education, occupation, and income level, we have examined the hazards associated with occupations in the lowest socioeconomic brackets. Another way to dramatize relationships between social status and longevity is to examine life expectancy in the uppermost echelons of society—the wealthy and the elite. Genetic endowment undoubtedly plays some role in their success, for it is often the extremely talented who rise to positions commanding power and fame. However, there is little doubt that their favored status with regard to life expectancy also results from the resources in their command which they can use to protect their health and the health of their families.

We have already noted that college graduates live longer than the general population, and among college graduates, those choosing occupations in education and religion stand out as long-lived. If you are a teacher or member of the clergy, your chances for a long life are excellent. We have also noted that the highest achievers among the college graduates live even longer than college graduates in general. These high achievers are the individuals selected into programs awarding advanced graduate degrees, and they are the individuals likely to be high achievers in any occupation they choose. Let us examine a few of the occupational categories into which these high achievers might fall.

Physicians

In the early 1940's Dr. L. I. Dublin and his associate noted that American physicians had only a slight advantage over the general population in terms of life expectancy at the beginning of their careers, and that after the age of 35, physicians had a somewhat shorter life expectancy than for white males in general. Compared to the mortality of men of equal social position, physicians had a much higher death rate. Dublin explained these data by suggesting that while doctors enjoy all the advantages of the professional group in terms of education, favorable home environment, high income, and excellent health care, they are under a great deal of stress and are exposed more to disease. Additionally, he found the suicide rate to be higher among physicians.

These factors appear to have less of an impact on physicians practicing in the 1970's, as Dr. L. J. Goodman recently reported that mortality rates among physicians are far lower than for the general population. He found that between the years of 1969 and 1973 the number of male physician deaths was only 75 percent of the expected deaths in the average white male population. Female physicians died at a higher rate than male physicians in relation to average American females (84 percent of the mortality rate of white females), but they were still dying at a rate lower than average. At all ages the mortality rate of physicians was better, particularly in New England and on the West Coast. Specialists had the lowest mortality rate among physicians. This may explain in part the difference between mortality rates of physicians in 1940 and 1970. There are far more specialists in the medical profession today than there were thirty years ago. Given that Dr. Dublin explained the higher death rate of physicians as resulting from stress, we might suspect that the general practitioner serving the needs of a large number of sick people in the whole range of age and ailment categories experiences more stress and is exposed to more health hazards than the specialist who lives longer.

Lawyers

The vocational risks to health incurred by physicians are totally absent in the case of lawyers who enjoy a long life expectancy due to their professional status and low-risk working conditions. Practicing law out of an office or in the courts among normally healthy people places the lawyer in a setting almost totally free from occupational hazards. The suicide rate in this occupational category is also low. Thus, the death rate among lawyers is considerably below that of the normal population.

Corporate Executives

Executives who have reached the highest levels in the business community also attain the most favorable conditions for longevity. In a study conducted over a 16-year period of more than 1,000 corporate executives of the 500 industrial corporations ranked by *Fortune* magazine as having the largest sales in the late 1950's, the Metropolitan Life Insurance Company found extremely low mortality rates. The rate was much lower than that for physicians, already a select group, in that it was only 63 percent of the mortality rate among white men in the general population. Comparable data for female corporate executives were not available because so few women had reached the top in these big corporations.

The favorable longevity is believed to reflect in physical and emotional fitness of these men for positions of responsibility. This may be because they are able to cope with and even thrive on stressful situations by harnessing tensions for productive use. It was concluded in this study of very successful businessmen that work satisfaction together with public recognition of accomplishments may well be an important determinant of health and longevity.

Other Elite Groups

In a study of more than 6,000 distinguished men listed in the 1950-51 edition of *Who's Who in America,* it was found that not only did these men outlive white American males in general, they also lived much longer than insured white American males, a group comprised mostly of middle and upper income level. Within the sample there was quite a difference in mortality among the different professions. While all of these eminent men lived longer than professional men in general, eminent correspondents and journalists had the shortest life span in the elite group, business executives were average, educators were among the longer lived of the elite, and the greatest longevity among the elite was experienced by the eminent scientists.

Men in high government positions as well as most other prominent men usually enjoy superior longevity. Dr. Joseph T. Freeman, a physician in Philadelphia, has compiled an impressive array of materials on the longevity of the elite, and he notes that state governors, members of Congress, members of the British House of Commons, United States Supreme Court Justices, and United States cabinet officers are among those eminent in government who live long. An exception to this rule is the case of American Presidents. Since the Civil War, Presidents of the United States from Lincoln to Johnson have experienced appreciably poorer longevity than did their contemporaries in the general population. (When the life expectancies of Presidents before the Civil War are included, however, Presidential life expectancy is longer than that for the average man.) The adverse impact on the longevity of recent U.S. Presidents may be associated with the awesome responsibilities associated with that possition. The relatively high number of Presidents assassinated during the period since the Civil War also dramatically shortened the life expectancy of the men as a group.

DOES RETIREMENT CAUSE DEATH?

Individuals of fame and eminence who live on average far longer than the general population are likely to be very involved in their profession and are able to pursue it in various ways as long as they wish. This is not the case for most people. Most of us, whether we like it or not, must give up our occupational role at the age of 65 because we are forced to retire. The identity and structure which working has given our lives are lost—and oftentimes so are we. Retirement is a stressful event for many and causes a dramatic change in lifestyle. Since societies fostering long life have nothing comparable to retirement, and since having a role in life and feeling useful and needed are characteristic qualities of those who have lived to be 100, many have speculated that mandatory retirement may contribute to shortening life expectancy.

There have been a number of studies comparing the mortality of older workers who stayed on the job to the mortality of those who retired. All of these studies, regardless of the occupation involved, demonstrated that life expectancy was shorter for the retired individuals. More of the retirees died, and right after retirement the death rate was particularly high. Thus, it became common in medical folklore to believe that an individual who was forced to retire would die much earlier than if he or she would be allowed to continue working. Retirement was seen as a stress which had deleterious physiological consequences which often proved fatal before the individual could adapt to the new lifestyle. The individual lost income, companionship, activity and stimulation, prestige, and identity, and these losses proved overwhelming.

While this retirement impact theory still has some adherants, it is generally believed that the studies demonstrating a relationship between retirement and death are seriously flawed because the health of the retirees was never considered. The reason most people retire early is because they are in poor health. They can no longer go on working. Thus, when you compare the life expectancy of these people who have retired due to poor health to the life expectancy of people who have been able to continue working, it is not surprising that the workers live longer. Retirement has been the *result* rather than the cause of poor health, and poor health results in an earlier death for the retirees. From the studies which have been carried out on retirement and longevity, there is no conclusive evidence that retirement causes death. It appears more likely that people who are nearer to death choose to retire—their poor health precluding them from working longer.

But what about those who are faced with mandatory retirement? Is it possible that they would live longer if allowed to continue in what they considered to be a productive work role? This is a question to which we do not have the answer, although some prominent longevity experts believe that retirement may cause early death. It is highly likely, however, that retirement has different effects on different kinds of people. Adjustment to retirement is associated with a number of variables, including income after retirement, health, and leisure activity. Other factors undoubtedly influencing how much of an impact retirement has on health and longevity are the degree to which a person derived his or her identity and enjoyment from the job and the number of interesting alternative hobbies and activities an individual has to occupy his or her time and interest after retirement. There may be some people who could be considered at high risk for health problems after retirement because their occupation was the center of their lives and their life outside the job was not very interesting to them. It has been shown that whitecollar workers find retirement more stressful immediately after they leave their job, but appear to adjust several years later, while bluecollar workers are happy to retire, but bored with retirement after several years. Thus, individual patterns may dispose some people to suffer after retirement—but it is just not clear that the difficulty in adjustment is stressful enough to cause death.

In recent years people seem to anticipate retirement and to plan for it. They are better prepared financially, their health is better in general, and they have developed leisure time hobbies and interests which carry them into retirement. More firms have established pre-retirement counseling and have prepared their employees and their families for the transition from work to leisure.

There is no question that people today anticipate retirement more than they have in the past because retirement has become more widespread. It is not clear, however, that people enjoy retiring any more in the 1970's than they did in earlier years. Indeed, many have fought mandatory retirement in the courts, and legislation against age discrimination has passed in Congress, paving the way for the eventual elimination of retirement on the basis of age. Legislation has already been proposed to make forced retirement illegal, and President Carter has indicated a willingness to sign such a bill. Thus, there are many who still view retirement as a stressful event and one which they want to avoid.

Given the need to make room for younger generations of workers and given the relatively high rate of unemployment in this country, it is unlikely that we will all be able to work into our 80's and 90's. On the other hand, schedules of part time work may be more common, and we may even develop a pattern of interspersing years of work with years of education and leisure through our adult lives. Such a pattern, in which no abrupt break is experienced at one single point in the life span, is more similar to the pattern experienced by long-lived peoples such as the Abkhasians.

While it is not clear that retirement leads to an earlier death, it is certain that having a meaningful, fulfilled life in the later years is associated with longer life. Thus, if we can develop a system—both as individuals and as a society—that provides for a meaningful and productive existence at all points of the life span, it will aid in our goal of extending human life to its maximum potential.

LIEESTYLE

12.
Geography, Climate, and Longevity

ᏞᏞOne of the most commonly held beliefs about long life is that there exists places in the world, usually kept hidden, where people live extraordinarily long. These Shangri-Las are often envisioned as valleys high in forbidding mountains where life is easy and food and beautiful scenery abound. Such a vision is not much different from the *hyperborean* myth discussed in Chapter 2. This involves the idea that somewhere in a far-away land there lives a people who enjoy perfect health and long life.

The search for climates and geographic locations ideal for longevity has been extensive and prolonged, but little has resulted. Dr. Zhores Medvedev, a Russian gerontologist, pointed out that the influence of special conditions in mountain areas, long believed to foster long life, have been ruled out. Super-longevous groups have been found in plains area as well as in the mountains in the U.S.S.R., and the climates in which long-lived people are found vary from tropical to extremely cold and dry. Indeed, climate appears to have almost nothing to do with longevity, and no climates have been found which are more conducive to long life. In the United States, you can live equally long in the heat of Texas, the drizzle of Oregon, the snow of Alaska, the dry, mountain air of Colorado, or the humid atmosphere of Louisiana. California sunshine has no more to do with long life than does Washington rain. The only climatic influences on longevity seem to be man-made. Climate can shorten life expectancy when it produces air inversions and lack of wind which exacerbate air pollution.

The case for geography as an influence on longevity is more promising because there are regional differences in life expectancy. The relationship does not appear to result from the terrain of the land, however, but from the lifestyle that arises as a result of geographic differences. The life of a farmer in the rural, flat country of the Middlewest U.S. appears to be the most conducive to longevity, while the life of a factory worker in the urban Northeast is about the least compatible with survival.

LONGEVITY PATTERNS IN THE UNITED STATES BY REGIONS, STATES, AND COUNTIES

An article published by the Metropolitan Life Insurance Company in 1976 began with the statement, "The average length of life continues to vary from one area of the country to another, particularly among white males, despite the long-term tendency for geographic mortality differentials to lessen." In Table 2 are the data reported in this article which are the life expectancies at birth and at ages 25 and 45 for white men and women in each of the fifty states. This table shows that states in the Midwest have the best longevity record in the country. North and South Dakota are the states which have the best life expectancy for men and women combined, and only a few states outside of the Midwest showed a greater life expectancy. The most hazardous states in terms of life expectancy are West Virginia and Nevada, followed closely by Alaska. Other high-risk states appear to be clustered on the Atlantic or Gulf coasts.

Because most states are large heterogeneous regions with a great mix of geographical areas and socioeconomic groups, epidemiologists have attempted to look at smaller units in order to get more clues about the causes of regional differences in longevity. Dr. H. I. Sauer and Dr. D. W. Parke studied the 25 highest and lowest death rate counties in the United States to get a notion of causal effects. Again, it is the counties in the Midwest which are most numerous among the low-mortality rate counties, while counties in the South and Northeast are most numerous among the high-risk counties.

In terms of the cause of death in the various counties, it appeared that natural causes as well as accidents and violence were much lower in low-risk than in high-risk counties. Stroke and hypertension, clearly stress-related diseases, were particularly high in the high-risk counties. Two-thirds of the high-risk counties also had very high rates for accidents and violence.

There were twelve factors implicated in longevity which differentiated the high and low-risk counties in Sauer and Parke's study. Low-risk counties showed a greater increase in their population than did high-risk counties, and there were also a greater percentage of people employed in construction. Both these factors indicate a faster growth rate for low-risk counties which were less densely populated and hence had more potential for growth. The percentage of older people in the population of low-risk countries was greater—probably as a direct consequence of the fact that the death rates for the age group between 35 and 74 were lower, leading more of this group to survive past the age of 65. More men over the age of 65 who were living at home (meaning not institutionalized) remained in the work force in the low-risk counties. This suggests that the older men were in better health because they could remain on the job. The different ethnic composition of the populations of high and low-risk counties was not considered to be a very important factor in the different mortality level, although it was noted that there are differences in longevity as a function of country of origin. People with Irish ancestors may live a shorter time than average, while people with ancestors from Norway, Sweden, Denmark, Germany, Italy, and the Netherlands may live slightly longer than average. Ireland also has a very high death rate, while the latter countries have low death rates. Nevertheless, compared with the marked geographic differences in death rates, death rates as a function of country of ancestry are very small. Many more of the low-death rate counties had a high proportion of farmers, and farming has been identified in some studies as the single occupation having the longest life expectancy. As noted earlier, mining and manufacturing are associated with shorter life, and counties in which more of the people were employed in these industries had higher death rates. Fewer females were employed in high-risk counties, again a sign of urbanization as was the population density. The more crowded counties had higher death rates.

Data from the Environmental Protection Agency indicated similar trends to the ones noted by Drs. Sauer and Parke. This agency indentified Hawaii as the healthiest place in the nation and Washington, D.C., as the unhealthiest. The clean air, absence of tension, slower pace, and absence of urban stresses makes most of Hawaii an ideal place in which to survive to a very old age. The urban, high-pressure, high crime, high cardiovascular disease rate in Washington, D.C., makes it a dangerous place to live.

RURAL VERSUS URBAN ENVIRONMENTS

The information regarding longevity as a function of region, state, and county point clearly to the fact that the biggest differences in longevity arise from living in rural as opposed to urban environments. The safest place to live in this country is in the country. This is neither a new discovery nor a recent phenomenon. Dr. George Gallup pointed out that well over a hundred years ago European physicians were aware of this fact. The following quotation was taken by Dr. Gallup from one of these physicians, Dr. Kitchiner, who said, "In Vienna, Berlin, Paris, and London the twentieth or twenty-third person died annually, while in the country around them, the proportion is only one in thirty or forty; in remote country villages, from one in forty to one in fifty—the smallest degree of human mortality on record is one in sixty." While the mortality rates today are far better than in Dr. Kitchiner's time, he still had identified a trend which has not yet been overcome by advances in medicine. Furthermore, Dr. Kitchiner was probably right about the causes of the mortality difference. He blamed "tensions and high living in the city—fear, grief and anxiety," as the causes for the differences. We might add to this list pollution, crime, crowding, lack of exercise and physical activity, and poverty.

TABLE 2. Expectation of Life, by State, 1969–1971 (White Males and Females, at Birth and at Age 25 and 45)

States by geographic division	Expectation of life, in years						Rank*					
	White male			White female			White male			White female		
	At birth	Age 25	Age 45	At birth	Age 25	Age 45	At birth	Age 25	Age 45	At birth	Age 25	Age 45
United States	67.9	45.7	27.5	75.5	52.4	33.5						
New England												
Maine	67.3	45.2	27.0	74.8	51.9	33.1	37	38	36	45	42	41
New Hampshire	67.5	45.3	26.9	75.2	52.1	33.1	34	33	39	37	37	43
Vermont	67.8	45.5	27.2	75.8	52.5	33.4	27	28	34	19	29	33
Massachusetts	68.3	45.7	27.3	75.6	52.3	33.4	16	23	30	27	33	32
Rhode Island	68.5	46.0	27.4	75.6	52.4	33.4	14	17	27	23	31	31
Connecticut	69.5	46.7	28.2	76.3	53.0	33.9	5	10	14	10	18	20
Middle Atlantic												
New York	68.0	45.6	27.4	74.9	51.8	32.9	20	26	29	43	47	48
New Jersey	68.6	46.0	27.5	75.2	51.9	32.9	11	18	24	39	44	47
Pennsylvania	67.7	45.3	26.9	74.7	51.5	32.6	29	34	40	48	48	49
East North Central												
Ohio	67.9	45.5	27.2	75.1	52.0	33.0	22	29	32	40	41	44
Indiana	67.7	45.5	27.2	75.2	52.2	33.3	32	30	31	36	34	38
Illinois	67.7	45.4	27.1	75.0	51.9	33.0	30	32	35	42	43	45
Michigan	68.0	45.8	27.4	75.2	52.2	33.3	21	22	28	35	35	37
Wisconsin	69.3	46.8	28.3	76.2	53.0	34.0	7	9	11	14	16	19
West North Central												

Minnesota	69.5	47.3	28.7	76.9	53.7	34.6	4	3	5	4	5	7
Iowa	68.9	46.8	28.4	76.6	53.6	34.6	10	8	10	8	7	8
Missouri	67.8	45.6	27.4	75.5	52.5	33.7	26	27	25	29	27	27
North Dakota	69.6	47.1	28.9	77.3	54.0	34.9	2	5	3	1	2	2
South Dakota	69.4	47.3	28.9	77.0	54.1	35.2	6	2	2	2	1	1
Nebraska	69.1	47.0	28.7	76.9	53.9	34.9	8	7	6	3	3	3
Kansas	69.1	47.0	28.6	76.8	53.7	34.8	9	6	8	5	4	4
South Atlantic												
Delaware	67.7	45.1	26.6	75.4	52.0	33.0	31	39	43	33	40	46
Maryland	67.8	45.3	26.9	75.4	52.1	33.1	25	36	41	30	38	39
District of Columbia	66.1	43.8	25.9	74.8	51.8	33.3	48	50	50	47	46	36
Virginia	67.7	45.3	27.0	75.7	52.7	33.7	28	35	37	20	24	28
West Virginia	65.8	44.1	26.4	74.0	51.3	32.5	51	48	48	49	50	50
North Carolina	66.8	44.6	26.6	75.7	52.8	33.9	40	43	44	21	21	22
South Carolina	66.1	43.8	25.9	74.8	51.9	33.1	47	51	51	46	45	40
Georgia	66.2	44.1	26.1	75.4	52.4	33.6	45	49	49	32	30	30
Florida	68.2	46.1	28.1	76.4	53.4	34.7	19	15	15	9	8	6
East South Central												
Kentucky	66.7	44.7	27.0	74.9	52.0	33.3	41	41	38	44	39	34
Tennessee	67.1	45.1	27.2	75.6	52.6	33.8	39	40	33	24	25	24
Alabama	66.6	44.6	26.8	75.6	52.8	33.9	42	44	42	22	22	21
Mississippi	66.1	44.3	26.6	75.3	52.5	33.7	46	47	46	34	26	25
West South Central												
Arkansas	67.6	45.7	27.7	76.3	53.3	34.5	33	25	22	11	11	10
Louisiana	66.6	44.4	26.4	75.2	52.1	33.3	43	46	47	38	36	35
Oklahoma	67.8	45.8	27.8	76.2	53.3	34.4	24	20	21	15	12	11
Texas	67.9	45.9	27.8	75.9	53.0	34.2	23	19	20	18	17	15

TABLE 2. (Continued)

States by geographic division	Expectation of life, in years						Rank*					
	White male			White female			White male			White female		
	At birth	Age 25	Age 45	At birth	Age 25	Age 45	At birth	Age 25	Age 45	At birth	Age 25	Age 45
Mountain												
Montana	67.2	45.7	27.9	75.6	52.9	34.1	38	24	17	28	19	17
Idaho	68.3	46.6	28.7	76.2	53.3	34.5	17	11	7	13	10	9
Wyoming	66.3	45.2	27.8	75.4	53.0	34.1	44	37	19	31	15	16
Colorado	68.5	46.5	28.5	76.0	53.2	34.3	12	12	9	16	14	14
New Mexico	67.3	45.8	28.3	75.1	52.4	33.6	36	21	12	41	32	29
Arizona	67.5	45.5	27.6	75.6	52.7	34.1	35	31	23	26	23	18
Utah	69.5	47.2	28.8	76.6	53.4	34.4	3	4	4	7	9	12
Nevada	66.0	44.5	26.6	73.7	51.1	32.5	50	45	45	51	51	51
Pacific												
Washington	68.3	46.1	27.8	76.0	52.8	33.9	18	16	18	17	20	23
Oregon	68.5	46.5	28.2	76.3	53.2	34.3	13	13	13	12	13	13
California	68.4	46.2	28.0	75.6	52.5	33.7	15	14	16	25	28	26
Alaska†	66.1	44.6	27.4	74.0	51.4	33.1	49	42	26	50	49	42
Hawaii†	71.0	48.5	30.1	76.8	53.6	34.7	1	1	1	6	6	5

* Rank determined by values computed to more than one decimal place.
† Relates to total males and females; values for the white population are not available.
SOURCE: National Center for Health Statistics, State Life Tables, 1969–1971. Reprinted from Metropolitan Life Insurance Company, "Longevity Patterns in the United States, Statistical Bulletin," 1976, 57, 2–4.

In Dr. Kitchiner's day, the mortality rate in the city was almost twice as great as in the country. This is no longer the case. Differences in life expectancy between rural and urban areas have been decreasing rather than increasing over the last century. The current rural-urban difference in life expectancy for both sexes is estimated at about two years, in favor of country dwellers.

The study of 402 people with an average age of 99 years carried out by Dr. George Gallup is in agreement with the statistics indicating that it is safer to live in the country. Fully 74 percent or almost three-fourths of Dr. Gallup's near-centenarians spent most of their lives on farms, in villages, or in small cities. Only 26 percent were residents of the larger urban areas most of their lives. Many of the people interviewed in this study lived within a mile of their place of birth. People in long-lived societies also tend to experience little change in their lives and remain in the small rural village or town from birth to old age. In this manner they avoid the stress of the unknown and the stress of leaving family and friends to establish a new life. This is an extremely rare phenomenon among contemporary Americans who move around the country at relatively frequent intervals, and who spend most of their lives in urban areas. Let us examine more closely the factors responsible for killing more Americans in the city.

HAZARDS IN THE URBAN ENVIRONMENT

Pollution

The clean, fresh air and blue sky of the country comes as a pleasant relief to urban dwellers used to burning eyes, soiled clothes and furnishings, and brown sky as a result of air pollution. What these city people may not recognize is that they are responding to a physiological benefit of the country air as well. A number of lines of research indicate that air pollution increases the risk of death. Thus, one reason that it is safer to live in the country is because industry and automobiles have not had as great an impact in polluting the air.

The injurious effects of breathing polluted air have been suspected since coal was introduced into the English economy in the early fourteenth century. It took several large scale disasters resulting from coal pollution before regulation was enacted. During the reign of Richard II (1377–1399) and under Henry V (1413–1422) steps were initiated to regulate the use of coal. Such steps were highly unsuccessful, however, and although warnings were issued throughout the ensuing centuries, little effort was made to reduce coal pollution. Thus, disasters such as the air pollution episode of 1909 which produced 1,063 deaths and the killing London smog of 1952 which claimed 4,000 lives were not avoided. Similar inaction has been the rule in the United States. One of the most highly polluted regions in our country is the Greater New York Area, and almost nothing was done to study or to control air pollution in this region until episodes in 1953, 1962, and 1966 prodded citizens into demanding government action.

From November 15 to November 24, 1953, a pattern of temperature inversions occurred in the New York City area which dramatically increased the intensity of air pollution. The daily death rate during that period was much greater than usual, and there was also a dramatic increase in clinic visits for upper respiratory and cardiac illnesses. Again from November 26 to December 6, 1962, sudden increases in daily death rate and in air pollution were recorded. An increase in the number of deaths in nursing homes was also observed during this period. In what has been called the Thanksgiving Day air pollution episode, a large mass of cold air moved over the Eastern seaboard on November 19, 1966, and lasted until November 25th. There was very little wind during this period, and pollution levels increased drastically. A number of significant health indices, including mortality rate, emergency room visits for respiratory complaints, and eye irritation, showed great increases until the wind blew away the high concentrations of irritants on the evening of November 25th. Late November appears to be a particularly dangerous time for pollution in New York City, and residents who make a habit of spending Thanksgiving with their family and friends in the country are protecting their health!

These brief episodes when air pollution is increased to unusually high levels dramatize the effect of pollution on longevity, but pollution takes its toll on health in far more subtle ways as well. These hazardous effects are less easily measured and sometimes they do not even appear with the measuring methods currently available. We are just beginning to recognize the disastrous effects.

Respiratory disease is one of the major negative effects of air pollution on health. A number of studies have demonstrated an increased incidence of respiratory disease among urban populations compared with that among rural populations. Many physicians concur with the general opinion that the Northeastern part of the United States can be considered the "sinus belt." Cancer, which has been associated with environmental pollution, also has a greater incidence in the city. Carbon monoxide, which is a major pollutant produced by automobile exhaust, has been shown to have significant negative effects on the nervous system and on the cardiovascular system. All of these effects have been shown to be exacerbated by the additional pollution experienced by smoking. Residents of the city who smoke compound the deleterious effects of living in a polluted environment. Few parts of the body escape the effects of pollution, and this makes the health of urban dwellers poorer than the health of inhabitants of rural areas who have the benefit of breathing clean air.

Psychological Stress Factors

The pace of life is faster in the city, and people feel more pressure in this kind of environment. In addition to pressures resulting from the job, the higher noise levels in the city and the density of the population produce psychological stress.

The peace and quiet enjoyed in the country is so dramatically different from the industrial and traffic noise of the city that many city dwellers take a few days to adjust to the quiet. Soon they have adapted so well to the absence of noise that the return to the city is jarring. Intense noise produces observable physiological damage to the ear, but the psychological damage which lower intensities of noise produce is more difficult to measure. Insomnia and irritability are two common complaints of individuals living in noisy environments. The relationship of these variables to stress factors which shorten life has not been documented, but we know that relaxation is conducive to long life. Living in a noisy environment does not help us to relax.

A number of studies have documented serious physiological consequences of over-crowding. When large numbers of animals are kept in relatively small cages they develop symptoms such as chronically elevated blood pressure, and they die at a younger age. Over-crowding is also stressful to humans, and it impairs their health.

That mental health is stressed to a greater degree in the city is suggested by the fact that more inner city residents than residents of the country seek help at mental health centers. Less is known about the mental health needs of rural populations, and fewer mental health services are available in rural areas. The stress of city life is enough to literally drive some people crazy. With others, it simply shortens their lives.

Lack of Physical Exercise

One of the probable reasons that farmers live longer is that they are active on the job and get a lot of physical exercise. Greater access to outdoor activities and more activity on the job are characteristics of living in rural areas. We have noted the physiological benefits of physical activity in Chapter 9. Active people have lower blood pressure and more efficient cardiovascular systems, and they are more relaxed. They also appear to live longer. In the city it is more difficult to exercise, and typical occupations in the city require inactivity. Furthermore, exercising in a polluted environment has mixed consequences. Some school systems in the Southern California area are so concerned about the harmful effects of strenuous exercise in heavy air pollution that they curtail the playground activity of children when pollution levels exceed specified standards. Thus, people in the country get more exercise, and they exercise in better environmental conditions.

Socioeconomic Status

More poor people are concentrated in the city than in the country. Although poverty certainly is not unknown in rural areas, it appears that poor people in the city have less access to resources which are conducive to long life. For example, there is less access to healthful food in the city where all foods must be purchased. In the country, vegetables and fruit can be grown. The jobs of poor city dwellers are more hazardous than low-paying jobs in the country as they involve laboring in industry where accidents and exposure to toxins increase the risk to survival. Crime rates are also higher in the city, and they are highest in areas where the poor live. Death by violence is greater among the lower classes, and poor people in the city are the most likely to be brutalized. All of these factors contribute to a higher mortality rate in urban areas where the poor are most concentrated.

Given the greater number of hazards to which urban inhabitants are exposed, it seems remarkable that the difference between life expectancy in rural and urban areas is only two years. One of the balancing factors is that the most modern medical facilities are located in the cities, and the ratio of physicians to patients is usually better in urban areas. Specialists who are highly skilled in the latest life-saving techniques most frequently work out of urban hospitals, and the equipment and technical support required to perform modern medical miracles is more likely to be found in urban hospitals. Added to this is the fact that Americans move their place of residence more frequently than people in any other country in the world. Migration between rural and urban areas is fairly high, and it is difficult to find people who have lived exclusively in one type of area. This is particularly true of suburban dwellers, who have some of the benefits of rural life along with some of the risks of the city. For this reason there has been somewhat of an equalization of life expectancy between geographic areas. However, we should not let this equalization dilute the impact of what we know about the benefits of rural life. Calm, quiet, peaceful, clean surroundings improve the quality of life. The more of us who can live in such environments, the greater our national life expectancy will be.

13.
Stress and Survival

ॐ»What would you consider to be a stressful event? Being involved in a car accident? Having a baby? Being fired? Most people would agree that all three events involve stress, but would you also consider working in a noisy office, taking a vacation, or changing your social activities stressful? Psychologists believe that any kind of change in life involves stress and adaptation. In addition, there are many aspects of the environment, particularly the urban environment, which are stressful. Indeed, life is full of stresses, and the essence of successful development and aging involves meeting and coping with stress.

Several life span developmental theories of personality center around the notion that successful adjustment involves mastering a series of stresses confronting the individual at various points in his or her life. These stressors have been called variously "psychosocial crises" and "developmental tasks." In young adulthood developmental tasks involve change and stress in that we must find and develop an intimate relationship with a mate, establish ourselves in an occupation, and bear and rear children. The stresses of middle age involve launching the children, establishing social and financial security, caring for aging parents, and adjusting to changing physical capacity and social status. In old age, change and stress are great as we face retirement, grief with the loss of friends and intimates, illness, and finally death. The point here is that stress is a part of life, and in living to be 100 the aim is not to avoid stress, but to learn how to cope with it effectively.

Scientists have a difficult time agreeing on what constitutes a stressor because the events perceived as stressful by one person may be seen as enjoyable by another. Even for the same individual, a similar event may be pleasant at one time and stressful at another time. Given the particular mood we are in and what we are doing at a given moment, we may hear birds singing and feel happy and uplifted or we may wish those damn birds would shut up! Some people find the pace and activity in New York City exhilarating while others are totally overwhelmed. Many individuals who become presidents and board directors of the largest corporations in the United States thrive on the challenges they face in the business world, while their colleagues suffer heart attacks and strokes from lesser responsibilities. A large part of stress is psychological. How we perceive and react to a given event can affect how long we live.

In response to stress, dramatic physiological changes take place. One of the first scientists to observe these changes was Dr. Walter B. Cannon, a Harvard physiologist, who measured various kinds of physiological responses in cats who were exposed to dogs. At the sight of the dog, adrenaline was released in the cat's bloodstream and one whole part of the nervous system, called the sympathetic nervous system, went into action. Increases in heart rate, circulation, and blood sugar levels occurred, blood-clotting mechanisms and breathing rate were accelerated, the senses became more keen and blood flow to the muscles was increased, while it decreased to systems not required at the moment such as the digestive system. All of these responses are adaptive, readying the cat for "fight or flight," as this response was named.

When the world was full of physical dangers, as it was when the human stress response evolved, it was tremendously adaptive for the body to mobilize in time of emergency. In modern life, however, it is rare that we face physical danger. Most of our stressors are mental, such as the shouts of the boss, an upcoming exam, or the cry of our child. The hormones released and the rapid changes in our vital functions which we experience in response to mental stress do not help us to escape the danger. Rather, the physiological responses which proved so adaptive to physical danger actually endanger our lives. In animals, severe stress produced experimentally leads to extensive damage of vital organs, and there are a number of human diseases resulting from stress which have similar serious consequences. High blood pressure or hypertension, kidney disease, and peptic ulcer are among the diseases called "stress diseases." We will see in Chapter 14 that the number one killer in the United States, heart disease, has also been related directly to the way an individual perceives and copes with stress. Emotions have direct physiological consequences which affect our health.

Why is it that there are so many stress diseases and that some people have heart attacks while others develop an ulcer? Part of the reason is that we all have inherited different constitutional make-ups, with differences in the organs which are vulnerable. Some of us secrete more stomach acid than others, making us prone to have ulcers. Others have weak respiratory systems, while still others have weak hearts and arteries prone to arteriosclerosis. Another reason that stress affects different organs systems in different individuals is that different stressors have different physiological consequences. For example, some situations make you depressed, which may affect your digestive system and your energy level. Other interactions may cause you to be frightened, embarrassed, or angry, in which case your heart pumps rapidly and you blush. Other confrontations may make your legs feel weak and cause you to be sick to the stomach. Thus, the same person may develop different symptoms depending on the source of the stress.

There are a number of ways to cope with stress. For one thing, it is important to keep yourself in good physical shape so that you will not be vulnerable to stress when it occurs. Shocking news which arrives the day after a wild party which left you with a hangover and too little sleep has a more devastating effect than if your body had received less abuse. We all know that worries which seem overwhelming when we are hungry or tired appear much more surmountable after we have eaten or slept. Proper diet, exercise, and sleep protect against vulnerability to stress. Another means to cope is to organize your life so that a number of stressful events do not occur together. While this is not always possible, there are a number of changes which we can control and which we may not always recognize as stressful, which have been shown to affect our health.

LIFE EVENTS AND YOUR HEALTH

Changes and stress have been discussed as factors central and even critical for life. However, in modern society, the pace of change and its resultant stress has been accelerated to the point where stress diseases are killing us more than any other thing. The accelerating rate of change and its consequences in our society have been extensively documented by Alvin Toffler in his book, *Future Shock*. He believes that this high level of change results in physiological and psychological distress because our ability to adapt and to make decisions is just swamped with too much overload. Other studies by physicians and professors have shown that physical illness is much more likely to occur after periods of rapid change in our lives.

A number of studies have extended and confirmed the finding that life changes preceded illness. In one study published in 1964, Dr. Richard Rahe, in collaboration with Dr. Thomas Holmes and other colleagues, examined life changes preceding five distinct health problems in seven different patient samples. Social changes in the year preceding the onset of the condition were greater than in any of the other ten years before the medical condition occurred. This was true for serious diseases such as heart disease and tuberculosis, and it also occurred for less serious medical problems such as skin disease and hernia. Even onset of pregnancy was related to life changes.

The first studies Drs. Holmes and Rahe carried out associating changes in life to illness involved interviewing patients who were hospitalized or who had suffered some change in health. The doctors asked these patients questions about what had happened to them over the previous years and found clustering of life change to precede a change in health. The second step in this research involved the development of a scale of life changes which could be used to identify persons at risk for health problems. Taking 43 events which they had identified from their clinical practice as being related to stress and illness, they asked a sample of close to 400 people to rate the life events according to how much readjustment each one acquired. The result was the "Social Readjustment Rating Scale," persented in Table 3.

The items on this scale are ranked according to how stressful each one was thought to be by a large number of people. Death of a spouse was considered to be the most stressful, requiring the most adjustment. The points (called "life crisis units" accorded to death of a spouse are 100, which is twice as many points as marriage, a life event rated by people as half as stressful. Likewise, being involved in minor violations of the law (such as getting a speeding ticket, jay walking, or disturbing the peace) was rated only 11 life crisis units, meaning that it is about a tenth as stressful as losing a spouse through death. Many different groups of people concur with this ranking system. There are no sex differences in rating, and people of different ages, different levels of education, different religions, and different races all are rather consistent in ranking these life events in terms of stress. Even people in different cultures (one study was carried out in Japan) seem to be in agreement as to the order of stressfulness of these life events.

The next step after developing a reliable measure of life change stress was to see if the scale could be used to predict illness. This was done by Dr. Rahe who studied illness patterns of 2,500 officers and enlisted men aboard three Navy cruisers. The men in the top third of the sample with regard to life change score developed nearly 90 percent more first illnesses during the first month of the cruise than the third with the lowest scores. Studies like this one helped Drs. Holmes and Rahe to develop the criteria determining how many points on the Social Readjustment Rating Scale were safe, and how many points put a person at risk.

Think about the changes which have occurred to you in the last year, and compute your own score on the Social Readjustment Rating Scale (Table 3). The total score involves the number of points you have accumulated over a one-year period. You get the number of life crisis units on the righthand column of the scale for each of the life event items on the lefthand column. Dr. Holmes gives the following example to show how the score is computed. He describes one year in the life of a singer who has just made it big, listing life crisis units (in parenthesis) for the various changes in the man's life.

As the royalties begin to roll in (38) from his first hit record (28), he decides that his image needs updating, so he buys a new wardrobe and lets his hair grow long (24). He begins to work longer and longer hours in the recording studio for his new album (20) and then departs for a three-month concert tour, staying in hotels and living out of a suitcase (25). He attends an endless string of parties and sees his old friends less and less (18). Concerts and parties keep him up most of the night, so he takes to sleeping in the daytime instead (16). He has to stay on a strict diet to avoid getting paunchy and has to give up his beloved chocolate eclairs altogether (15). Whereas he used to play tennis twice a week and go sailing on week ends, now the most exercise he gets is tuning his guitar (19). His wife, initially delighted at the new excitement, finds she is really not a part of his new life, despite the fact that they have moved (20) into a new home. The couple argue more and more (35) about the time he spends away from home and their sexual relationship deteriorates (39).

The singer has accumulated 297 points in a short period of time. If his wife now begins seeing a psychiatrist (44) and files for a legal separation (65), he will find himself firmly in a position of high risk for experiencing some major change in health. In his particular profession alcoholism or other heavy drug use might be a likely possibility, but he might just as easily develop a bleeding ulcer or fall off the stage one night and break his leg.

Just as Dr. Holmes has done, be sure to compute all of the changes which occurred over the past year. Many of them will have been pleasant and will not have caused you worry. Thus, you might be reluctant to consider them stressful. Nevertheless, any kind of change appears to be associated with stress and with increasing the individual's chance of developing health complications. All different kinds of health conditions may occur from serious to minor diseases, to auto or other accidents, to the need for surgery, to a suicide attempt.

TABLE 3 The Social Readjustment Rating Scale

Rank	Crisis	Life crisis unit	Your score
1	Death of spouse	100	_____
2	Divorce	73	_____
3	Marital separation	65	_____
4	Jail term	63	_____
5	Death of close family member	63	_____
6	Personal injury or illness	53	_____
7	Marriage	50	_____
8	Fired from work	47	_____
9	Marital reconciliation	45	_____
10	Retirement	45	_____
11	Change in family member's health	44	_____
12	Pregnancy	40	_____
13	Sex difficulties	39	_____
14	Gain of new family member	39	_____
15	Business readjustment	39	_____
16	Change in financial state	38	_____
17	Death of a close friend	37	_____
18	Change to different line of work	36	_____
19	Change in number of arguments with spouse	35	_____
20	Mortgage over $10,000	31	_____
21	Foreclosure of mortgage or loan	30	_____
22	Change in responsibilities at work	29	_____
23	Son or daughter leaving home	29	_____
24	Trouble with in-laws	29	_____
25	Outstanding personal achievement	28	_____
26	Spouse begins or stops work	26	_____
27	Begin or end school	26	_____
28	Change in living conditions	25	_____
29	Revision of personal habits	24	_____
30	Trouble with boss	23	_____
31	Change in work hours or conditions	20	_____
32	Change in residence	20	_____
33	Change in schools	20	_____
34	Change in recreational habits	19	_____
35	Change in church activities	19	_____
36	Change in social activities	18	_____
37	Mortgage or loan less than $10,000	17	_____

38	Change in sleeping habits	16	_____
39	Change in number of family gatherings	15	_____
40	Change in eating habits	15	_____
41	Vacation	13	_____
42	Christmas season	12	_____
43	Minor violation of the law	11	_____
Total			_____

SOURCE: T. H. Holmes and R. H. Rahe, "The Social Readjustment Rating Scale," *Journal of Psychosomatic Research*, 1967, 11, 213–218.

Once you have totaled your points for the year, you can interpret them in the following manner. A score below 150 points is considered safe. Your chances for a serious health change in the next two years is about 33 percent based on estimates for average risk to health in the United States. If you scored between 150 and 300 points, the chance you are risking a serious health problem rises to 50 percent. A score of 300 or more points puts you in the high-risk category. People scoring this high have a 90 percent chance of having a serious health change in the next couple of years. If you are in this high-risk category, you should take particularly good care of yourself, try to avoid any further changes for the next year or so, and consult with your physician at the least indication of illness.

While life change is something we cannot and should not avoid, we should attempt to manage our lives in such a way as to minimize the number of changes occurring all at once. We know in advance when many of the major changes listed on the Social Readjustment Rating Scale will occur, and we can plan for them and avoid making them more stressful by accompanying them with additional unnecessary changes. For example, if you are planning to get married, that is not the time to think about changing jobs. Right after a divorce, try to maintain some stability in your life by maintaining your old sleeping and eating habits, your same work habits, and good relations with your boss. That this is difficult and that divorce and death of a spouse are two of life's most stressful and health-threatening events have been independently confirmed by statistics indicating the higher rate of illness and employee absenteeism in divorced and widowed individuals along with the higher death rate in these two groups. This leads us to consideration of the stress-reducing effects of marriage and the stress-producing effects of loss of spouse through divorce or death.

STRESS AND MARITAL STATUS

United States Public Health Service statistics demonstrate that regardless of sex or race, death rates are lower for individuals who are married than for those who are single, widowed, or divorced at every age past 20. The highest death rates at every age after 24 occur in people who are divorced. Formerly married persons, including widowed, divorced, and separated individuals, also have higher rates of physical and mental illness and physical disability than do married people. Higher physical illness and disability rate is not a greater problem for those who are single, although they have higher mental illness, suicide, homicide and accident rates.

There seem to be three general explanations for lower death, illness, accident, and homicide rates in those who are married. First of all, marriage is selective in that people who have chronic health conditions or serious disabilities, or who suffer from generally poor health are less likely to get married. This is a selection factor. The healthiest, the ones most likely to survive the longest, are the individuals selected for marriage. From this perspective, marriage is not adding to the life expectancy of people. Those who would under any circumstances live a long time are the people who get married. Marriage is associated with long life, but it is not causing it.

Another reason that the statistics indicate that married people live longer may be because marriage is the norm in our society and those who do not get married are considered abnormal. Being in an abnormal social group is stressful, and it can wear a person down and make him or her more prone to illness, accidents, and crime. That many more people are remaining single or becoming single again as a result of divorce is having an effect on the social status of being single. It is not as stigmatizing in the 1970's to be single as it was in the 1950's. Thus, one of the potential causes of mortality differences between single and married people, the social pressure and stress experienced by the unmarried or formerly married, may be decreasing. This may cause a reduction in the difference in life expectancy between married and unmarried people.

The third explanation put forward to account for health and mortality differences between the married and unmarried is that marriage has life-sustaining effects. The intimacy and close interpersonal ties fostered by marriage help individuals to maintain a sense of well-being. People who are happier live longer, and marriage often creates happiness and contentment.

One of the key factors leading marriage to cause longer life appears to be the social ties and social status it confers. This was shown by two sociologists from Brown University, Drs. Frances Kobrin and Gerry Hendershot. They reasoned that if social ties are an important concomitant of longevity, than nonmarried people with greater social ties should live longer than nonmarried people who are alone. They examined the living arrangements of a national cross section of people who had died between the ages of 35 and 74, and found that for both men and women, living with other people, particularly close relatives, added years to life. Among nonmarried men, those who served as the head of the family lived longest, and those living with families, even when they were not the head, lived longer than nonmarried men who lived alone. The mortality rate for nonmarried men living alone was extremely high.

In women, the situation was slightly different. Nonmarried women who were the head of a household lived the longest of all nonmarried women, but living alone was better for women than living in a family in which they were not the head. Perhaps women living alone are better able to maintain intimate ties to family and friends than are men who live alone.

Physiological differences between people without close social ties have been found by Dr. John Cassel of the University of North Carolina. Dr. Cassel's work was reported by Kenneth Lamott in his book, *Escape from Stress: How to Stop Killing.* This research suggests that there are marked changes in the hormone levels of people deprived of warm social ties and social approval, and that this makes them more vulnerable to disease. Dr. Cassel feels that these results may explain why the death rate from heart disease, cancer, and strokes is greater in big cities than in other parts of the country. Many more people are alone in the city than in the suburbs or in rural areas where people tend to live in families.

In addition to the benefits of warm, physical and emotional ties, living with another person helps to regulate life and to facilitate good health practices. When you live alone you are much less likely to cook a meal for yourself or to eat nutritiously at regular hours. If you are sick, you may wait longer to go to the doctor, and there is no one at home to nurse you back to health. Married people visit physicians and clinics more frequently, but their average hospital stay is shorter. They practice preventative medicine. More of the people who live alone are in the low financial brackets as well. Thus, they are less able to afford good food and adequate medical care. Single and formerly married people also have less health insurance. Being married helps one to avoid these obstacles to good health and stimulates spouses to take care of themselves and of one another. That married people are in better health and take better care of themselves adds to their life expectancy causing a gap between the life expectancy of married and nonmarried people. That divorced and widowed individuals commit suicide in much greater numbers than any other population group and that the recently widowed often die because they no longer have the will to live makes the gap in longevity between married and nonmarried individuals even greater. Single and formerly married people also have a higher mortality rate due to accidents and homicide.

A study of suicides by marital status shows that the rates are lower for married people than for single, widowed, or divorced people in all age groups except the very young and the very old. Divorced people have the highest rates, which are three to five times as great as the rates of married people under 65. Accidental death—which in instances such as motor vehicle accidents involving only one car, drownings, poisonings, and falls may be suicide—is also much higher among single, widowed, and divorced people. It seems that people who are isolated and alone experience stress as more painful than those who live with others in intimate relationships. Furthermore, the stress of the separation itself, particularly in the case of losing a spouse through death, can be fatal.

In an exhaustive review of the literature on the loss of a significant other as a predictor of death, Dr. Kay F. Rowland of the University of California at Los Angeles concluded that death often results from the loss of a spouse. Dr. Rowland argued that the most convincing evidence came from studies in which recently bereaved were followed for a period of years after the death of their spouse. The mortality rate in these people was much greater than it was in people matched for age and health status who had not lost their spouse. The death rate for the bereaved was greatest in the first six to twelve months following bereavement. After this period the mortality rate returned gradually to the level of married people. The loss of a spouse appeared to be most stressful for men, who died at a greater rate than women during bereavement. There is also some evidence that loss of a parent or sibling results in an increase in mortality among close family members. The loss of close emotional ties appears to be the most stressful event we can experience as humans, and if we have not developed other relationships and activities which can sustain us over this difficult period, we may not be able to adapt to the change.

A study of the effects of loss of intimate personal relationships due to death or divorce suggests how that loss is best survived. The important element in survival and continued satisfaction in life seems to be the development or maintenance of other close personal ties. The strategy used by people who cope successfully with stress is to develop a network of friends who stand by them and support them during their time of need. Isolation and loneliness are the worst consequences of separation from loved ones, and it is essential to avoid being alone during this time. If you are a friend of someone who has recently separated or been widowed, spend some time with them and give them affection and support. If you are yourself recently separated or widowed, don't bear your grief alone. Gather your family and friends around you and let them help you in this time of stress. Don't wall yourself off emotionally or refuse to let people come close. You'll be depriving yourself of the very thing which can sustain you through this difficult period.

Psychologists have found that it is particularly effective in the case of widowhood to bring together those who have recently lost a spouse to encourage them to discuss their feelings and their loss. No one can fully understand the profound sadness which must accompany the loss of a life-long partner unless he or she has experienced it. Thus, letting the bereaved be a comfort to one-another provides them with a source of great understanding and with the potential for the development of new personal ties.

Friends buttress the stressful effect of any kind of loss, and one of the outstanding qualities of centenarians is that they love people and have spent much of their lives fostering close friendships. A series of studies carried out by Marjorie Lowenthal and her colleagues at the University of California at San Francisco have demonstrated that life satisfaction in old age is greatest when a person has at least one close, intimate friend. Professor Lowenthal calls this person a confidant. It can be a friend or a spouse, and usually it is a person of the same generation who is familiar with the world the friend has known. Such a person can be of the same or of the opposite sex. The important ingredient in the relationship appears to be the ability to open up and expose the details of your life. Intimacy and personal closeness provide an emotional cushioning, particularly in time of crisis and stress. Thus, an important ingredient in longevity is friendship. Take time with your friends and make sure you have a few who are more than just acquaintances. Such friendships make life more enjoyable—and they provide for adaptation and survival in the face of adversity.

ENVIRONMENTAL STRESSORS AND THEIR CONTROL

Totally apart from human interaction, stress can come from the physical environment and from changes in the environment. Most stresses in the environment are not so intense that they produce immediate physical damage. The damage is cumulative, such as the respiratory ailments resulting from continuous exposure to air pollution. Another example of the cumulative effect is psychological damage wrought by noise or crowding which may lead to stress diseases such as hypertension.

Dr. Jerome Singer of the State University of New York at Stony Brook and Dr. David Glass of the University of Texas at Austin have studied the long term effects of urban stress, and they believe that there are three general characteristics affecting the experience of stress. After-effects of stress are tremendously influenced by the predictability of the stressor. If its onset is preceded by a signal or if it occurs at predictable times, its effect will be much less. An example of this is seen in people who live near railroad tracks where the trains keep a regular schedule. Soon these people do not notice the trains, and are surprised when visiting guests find the noise annoying. Indeed, research measuring the response of the brain to predictable events has shown that brain activity habituates, that it is decreased or almost disappears when stimuli are presented over and over again. The brain adapts to the predictable, and it responds dramatically only when the rate is changed or when the predicted stimulus is absent.

A second factor affecting the stress experience is the social context in which the stress occurs. The noise of the neighbor children is much more annoying to a grandparent than the noise of the grandchildren. We are willing to tolerate and even enjoy certain phenomena if they occur under one set of conditions while we find the same phenomena aversive at another time or place.

The most important factor is the feeling of control. When people feel that they have choices in a situation or that they can escape from the stressor, it has far less effect on them than when they don't have the feeling of control. Control has been shown to be especially critical to survival in one type of environmental stress—moving older people who live in nursing homes. A number of studies have shown that the elderly die at excessively high rates in the first year after moving into a nursing home or after they have been moved from one nursing home to another. That many of these people would not have died if they had not been moved has been demonstrated by comparing the mortality rates of those moved to those in equally poor health who were not moved. The individuals remaining in the familiar environment survived in greater numbers. Giving these people some feeling of control over the impending move also improves survival rate. This has been shown independently in a number of studies in which elderly patients who had to be relocated were told six months in advance about the move and the staff moved with them. Taking these precautions, there was no increase in the mortality rate after the patients were moved.

COPING WITH STRESS

We have already seen that developing a network of friends and fostering a few close, intimate relationships are ways to protect yourself from being overwhelmed by stress. Another coping mechanism is to arrange situations so that you can control the stress. Even if you choose not to exercise the control, the consequences of stress over which you have control are less. Several other means to reduce the effects of stress are to place the stress in a favorable context and to regulate your environment so that the stress is predictable. Convince yourself that the source of the stress is necessary or useful or arrange your schedule to fit the occurrences of the stress. For example, if there is road construction on your route to work, consider how good the highway will be when the work is done, or take an alternate route, or go in at a different time to avoid the hassle.

A very important response to learn in the face of stress is to relax. If you can condition your body to unlearn the "fight or flight" response of mobilization (the racing pulse, the sweaty palms, the tenseness in the back and neck muscles), and instead respond with relaxation to stressful events, you will save your body years of wear and tear. Relaxation techniques are used by many clinicians to help patients surmount their problems. First they learn to relax, then they learn to think about a stressful thing or event while they are relaxed, and finally they learn to relax in the presence of the stressful stimulus. Many phobias are cured in this manner, and this technique has also been used to combat general anxiety and tension and even to decondition patients who have behavior patterns which make them prone to heart attack.

Drs. Gay Luce and Erik Peper, experts on relaxation techniques, prescribe these exercises to reduce stress. These exercises will help you to become familiar with tension and relaxation in your body. Get rid of tight clothes, your watch, and even your glasses before you begin. Sit on the edge of a straight chair (wooden, if possible) with your knees about 12 inches apart and your legs slanting forward. First sit up very straight. Then let yourself collapse like a rag doll. Your head should hang forward, your spine should be rounded, and your hands should rest on your knees. Once you are comfortable, start talking to yourself, saying, "My right arm is heavy, my right arm is heavy. . . ." Concentrate on your arm from the tips of your fingers to your armpits, and repeat the words for about seconds. When your arm is really heavy, make a fist, flex your arm, take a deep breath and open your eyes. Repeat the whole procedure three or four times a day, it only takes 30 seconds, and work at it until you are really successful in making your right arm feel very heavy. After you can control your right arm in this manner, work on your left arm, on your right and left leg, and on your head, neck and torso until you can relax in this manner from head to toe.

Relaxation is not easy. It takes concentration, effort, and a lot of practice, but you may be surprised at how well the effort pays off. You may experience more energy and greater efficiency in your thinking when you learn to reduce tension and relax.

Another type of relaxation exercise involves breathing. Relaxed breathing, practiced in quiet moments and applied throughout the day in all of your activities can help alleviate tension. Think about your breathing when you do the following exercises, and try not to think of other things. Make breathing pleasurable, and do the specific exercises at least twice a day with a loose belt and a relaxed stomach.

Lie on your back on the floor with a pillow under your head. Your knees should be bent, with your feet on the floor about 8 inches apart. Make sure that your spine is straight. Put one hand on your stomach and the other on your chest. Take deep breaths into your stomach and feel it rise. Your chest should hardly move at all. Do this until it becomes easy. Then do the following: smile slightly, breathe in through your nose and out through your mouth, blowing with a slight whistling sound, like the wind. Your jaw, tongue, and mouth should be dropped slightly, and relaxed. Think about the sound and the feeling of the breathing, taking long, slow breaths which make your stomach move. Do this for five to ten minutes at a time.

Another breathing exercise requiring even less effort is to sigh deeply, making a sound of deep relief. Let all of the air out of your lungs and then just let the air come back in. Don't force inhaling—let the air come in naturally. Repeat this ten times.

Be sure not to force your breathing with these exercises. Otherwise you will hyperventilate and begin to feel dizzy. Breathe at a natural rate. Try to determine your natural rate and flow with it. It may help to follow your breath in your mind. Pretend you can see it entering your nose and throat and flowing to your lungs and diaphragm, pushing up your stomach. Think of it as reaching all parts of your body through your blood and touching and relaxing you as you inhale—leaving you composed and serene as you exhale.

After you have become comfortable with breathing so that your stomach moves, practice it at odd moments during the day when you are sitting or standing. Direct all of your attention to the breathing and to the feeling of relaxation it gives you. When you know how to relax yourself by breathing in this fashion, start practicing it every time you feel yourself getting tense. This can be as simple as concentrating on breathing when the car in front of you is moving too slowly. Then you can escalate your relaxation therapy to interpersonal encounters. Try it when you start to get irritated with your spouse or family, or when someone at work annoys or frustrates you.

In addition to these physical exercises, you may want to meditate for fifteen to thirty minutes a day as a form of relaxing your mind. One way to do this is to chant to yourself. Choose a word that is pleasant like "peace" or "love" and say it first out loud so that you can hear it and then mentally to yourself. Sit and listen to the mental repetition of the chant, and when your mind starts to wander to other thoughts, gently bring it back to the chant. You may not notice any effect for several weeks, but if you stay with meditation for several months, the results it will bring you may be surprising.

Another type of meditation which involves visual imagery can be carried out twice a day for ten-minute periods. Pick a favorite object, such as a flower, and think about it and picture it. Gently bring your thoughts back to the object when they stray—just enjoy the object. Use the object in stressful moments to calm your mind. Such contemplation can be carried out for a few minutes even at your desk during a break, and it can provide you with far more uplift than a cup of coffee. Be prepared to practice it a while before feeling the results, however. Relaxation is a process of slowing down—and part of the slowing involves developing the patience and calm to detect the subtle and extremely rewarding changes it can produce.

14.

Personality
and Long Life

&If you have had the pleasure of interacting with a number of those who have lived to be 90 or 100 you were probably struck by the characteristic calm and serenity which marks these people. The one stereotype most common in all very long-lived individuals is that they are happy. In their old age they continue to have a purpose in life and feel needed. They have confidence in themselves, and they generally enjoy life. Absent in these individuals is anger, depression, or hostility. Rather, they consider themselves cheerful and easygoing. They have made time to enjoy people and the simple pleasures and beauty in life.

In his interviews of near-centenarians, Dr. George Gallup found them to be a happy, well-adjusted group. Sixty-eight percent described themselves as cheerful. A majority (58 percent) said that they were easygoing, hard to provoke (61 percent), and that they liked to take things as they come (65 percent). Most of them (57 percent) believed that it was difficult for someone to hurt their feelings, indicating that they were self-confident. A remarkable 84 percent of these long-lived individuals felt that their lives had been well-spent. They were satisfied with the way they had lived their lives.

On six questions regarding happiness, these older individuals generally presented a very positive picture. Compare your own personal happiness to that expressed by people successful at long life to determine how much your own pattern fits theirs. (See Table 4.)

Although many of the long-lived people in Dr. Gallup's sample were successful in their occupations, they were not driven by their ambitions. The aggressive, perfectionistic, driving personality characteristic of so many upwardly striving Americans was not part of the pattern observed in the successfully long-lived. The famous University of Chicago football coach, Amos Alonzo Stagg, one of the most respected individuals ever to succeed in that high-pressure profession, provides an ideal example of the calm, confident manner in which longevous people manage their careers. Dr. Gallup quotes Alonzo Stagg about his approach to life: "I've known lots of coaches who couldn't eat before a game, but I've never missed a pre-game meal in my life." Defeat did not disturb Alonzo Stagg: "My main concern was for the boys. I wanted them to produce as best they could with fair methods and sportsmanship. If we lost, I didn't take it to heart. I wasn't afraid of losing my job. I did my coaching on the field, and gave lots of vitality to it. But when the day was over, I didn't bring it home with me. I didn't worry over it."[1] Amos Alonzo Stagg lived to be 102 years old.

Contrasted to Coach Stagg are the countless tens of thousands of Americans who mindlessly push themselves to achieve at an increasingly pressured, frenzied pace. The pressure at the office overflows to the home and family life, which becomes subordinate to the demands of the occupation. The simple pleasures of life are ignored in the face of what is considered more important—success and higher income. This personality syndrome has been identified and described by Drs. Meyer Friedman and Ray Rosenman, cardiologists in medical practice in San Francisco, as the Type A pattern. Drs. Friedman and Rosenman have argued persuasively that this Type A personality pattern more than any other single factor in American life predisposes an individual to heart attack.

TABLE 4 The Happy Lives of the Oldsters as Indicated in Their Answers to Six Important Questions[2]

In general, would you say that throughout your lifetime, you have been:

Very happy	53%
Fairly happy	42%
Not so happy	4%
Don't know	1%

What do you think was the happiest period of your life?

Childhood	6%
Teens	5%
When first married	15%
While children growing up	13%
After children grown up	10%
Married life	12%
Old age	4%
No specific period stated	35%

Has your home life been peaceful and quiet?

Yes	94%
No	3%
Don't know	3%

Looking back over your life, were you the type of person who preferred to have people around or have you gotten more pleasure from being alone?

Preferred people around	84%
More pleasure from being alone	11%
Don't know	5%

How would you describe your married life?

Extremely happy	52%
Fairly happy	31%
Not so happy	5%
No answer	4%
Never married	8%

Would you say that you have had a happier life than most of your friends?

Yes	40%
The same	35%
No	6%
Don't know	19%

SOURCE: G. Gallup and E. Hill, "The Secrets of Long Life," (New York: Bernard Geis Associates, 1960), (pp. 139–140). Reprinted with the permission of the publisher, Bernard Geis Associates, Inc. © 1960 by George Gallup and Evan Hill. © 1959 by The Curtis Publishing Company.

TYPE A PERSONALITY AND SURVIVAL

"We believe that the major cause of coronary artery and heart disease is a complex of emotional reactions, which we have designated Type A Behavior Pattern," state Drs. Friedman and Rosenman. In their book, *Type A Behavior and Your Heart*, these cardiologists present the evidence, research, and treatment of this problem in which they have been involved for the past twenty years.

Working together in a busy cardiology practice, these physicians, like most of their colleagues at the time, focused on the traditional predictors of cardiovascular disease—high cholesterol level, high blood pressure, smoking, and obesity. Friedman and Rosenman admit that it took them years to become aware that these health factors alone could not explain their patients' illness. One clue they overlooked until long after it was presented was provided by an upholsterer. He was employed by the doctors to fix the seats of the chairs in their reception room. The upholsterer was curious about what kind of a practice the cardiologists had because he could not understand why only the front edge of their chair seats were worn out. Apparently the cardiologists' patients seldom sat back in the chairs.

Another curious phenomenon noted by Friedman and Rosenman was that although high cholesterol level predicted the onset of coronary heart disease, the diets of their patients did not always include a high fat and high cholesterol content. Furthermore, the doctors were aware of many individuals ingesting a lot of fat and cholesterol who neither developed a high level of cholesterol in their blood nor had any symptoms of heart disease. To study this phenomenon more carefully they investigated the dietary habits of volunteers from the San Francisco Junior League and their husbands. Since American white women develop coronary heart disease much less frequently than American men, the cardiologists expected that the women's diet would include much less cholesterol and animal fat. This was not the case. The diets of the successful business and profession men and their wives who were in the Junior League were almost identical. While many believed that hormonal differences between men and women caused women to be less prone to coronary heart disease, Drs. Friedman and Rosenman did not favor this hypothesis. They felt instead that the women led less stress-producing lives and dealt with stress in a more effective manner than their husbands. When the female participants were asked why so many of their husbands were having heart attacks, the women were absolutely certain that diet was not involved. The women firmly believed that the stress related to their husbands' jobs was killing them.

While skeptical of any diagnosis suggested by untrained lay people, the physicians nevertheless decided to pursue this lead. They did so by sending a questionnaire to 150 businessmen involved in the industrial and commercial community of San Francisco, asking them to chose from a number of items what they felt had caused a friend's recent heart attack. More than 70 percent of these businessmen believed that excessive competitive drive and the need to meet deadlines was the outstanding characteristic of heart attack prone people. Less than 5 percent believed that a diet excessive in fatty or high cholesterol foods or cigarette smoking, or lack of exercise was responsible for heart attacks. In addition to the laymen's opinion, Drs. Friedman and Rosenman solicited the opinions of 100 internists who treated coronary patients. This group confirmed the opinions of the Junior League women and the 150 businessmen. They, too, believed that the phenomenon most likely to precede a heart attack was excessive competitive drive and the need to meet deadlines.

From a contemporary perspective such responses are not seen as particularly surprising, but in the late 1950's when these studies were conducted, the medical journals were replete with articles stressing the significance of diet, exercise, and cigarette smoking in the etiology of heart disease. While these factors are of major import, another significant factor, the personality factor, was almost totally ignored in the medical literature. Cardiologists were treating the habits rather than the personality of the individuals developing heart disease.

Drs. Friedman and Rosenman set out at this point to determine the total personality pattern related to heart disease. They came to call it the Type A Behavior Pattern, and saw as its central characteristics the constant feeling of time urgency coupled with excessive competitive drive. With this beginning pattern, they undertook biochemical and epidemiological studies to determine all of the traits involved in the Type A personality and to investigate the role of the pattern in the development of heart disease.

One of the first steps was to find individuals who were free from coronary heart disease but possessing the Type A Behavior Pattern. The doctors predicted that these individuals would show some of the biochemical abnormalities present in coronary patients. Thus, they got a sample of men identified as in good health but possessing an intense sense of time urgency and a strongly developed competitive drive. It turned out that the men with the strong competitive drive also often gave evidence of easily aroused hostility. Twelve years later these men were still being studied by Drs. Friedman and Rosenman. Results showed that serum cholesterol level often varied directly with the intensity of the Type A Behavior Pattern. For example, in a group of accountants the cholesterol level rose from January to April, and by the April 15th tax deadline, both the accountants' sense of time urgency and their cholesterol level reached a peak. By May and June, when the deadline had passed and the sense of time urgency had waned to almost nothing, cholesterol levels fell. That the changes in cholesterol level were due to the stress was inferred because nothing else in the lives of these men changed over the six months during which they were followed. Their diet, smoking, and exercise habits remained essentially the same.

Following up on this work in various other studies, Friedman and Rosenman found that individuals exhibiting extreme forms of the Type A personality had every blood fat and hormone abnormality found in the majority of coronary patients. It appeared that the behavior patterns of Type A people were causing them to have coronary heart disease. In eighty 35 to 60-year-old men who had been selected to characterize the highly aggressive, competitive, time pressured pattern, a higher serum cholesterol level was found than in eighty men of the same age who were relaxed about deadlines and who were not terribly competitive. Furthermore, in 28 percent of the seemingly healthy Type A men, coronary heart disease had already developed. They had seven times as much heart disease as the men in the more relaxed group, yet the diets and exercise patterns of the two groups were almost identical.

These results were replicated in women. Aggressive, excessively competitive, time-pressured women had much higher serum cholesterol levels than their calmer, less driven counterparts. However, it was more difficult to find Type A women than Type A men. Most women were more in touch with their feelings and less driven by time. While this was true of women in the early 1960's, it may be less true today. As more and more women aspire to successful careers, they too, may become more victimized by the Type A pattern.

Expanding their approach, Friedman and Rosenman initiated a study of over 3500 healthy men enlisted from large corporations in the San Francisco area. These men were classified according to behavior pattern and given physical examinations. Ten years later, over 250 of these men had suffered coronary heart disease. The single best predictor of heart attack was Type A behavior pattern. Those exhibiting the pattern at the beginning of the study were almost three times more likely to develop heart disease in the next ten years than individuals classified as having a Type B Behavior Pattern. Type B individuals were free from time pressure and hostility and were not willing to chain their lives to their careers. Risk factors in heart disease such as weight, diet, and moderate smoking did not predict heart disease in Type B individuals, for no matter what their habits, they seemed immune to heart attack. The fact that most of them did not smoke and maintained reasonable health habits was an additional protection to the Type B's. While the major predictors of heart attack such as high blood pressure, diabetes, high blood cholesterol level, and heavy smoking did predict the disease in Friedman and Rosenman's sample, they predicted no better than Type A pattern. Unfortunately, many of the men showing the Type A pattern also smoked in excess and had high blood pressure. Neither of these risk factors was present in most of the Type B men.

All of these correlational studies by Friedman and Rosenman were highly suggestive of a strong relationship between the Type A pattern and heart disease, but it had been impossible to experimentally manipulate personality to show it caused heart disease. With only the evidence from human studies, the doctors could not rule out the possibility that some hereditary or environmental factor caused both the Type A personality and the heart disease. If that were the case, then treating the personality would not benefit the patients because the Type A personality would not be causing the disease. To demonstrate a causal relationship between aggressive personality and factors causal in heart disease, the cardiologists undertook studies in rats. By damaging the hypothalamus, a center buried deep in the brain which regulates vital functions such as breathing, temperature, and heart rate as well as being involved in the regulation of emotions, the researchers were able to make rats develop aggressive, hostile, competitive personality patterns. Gentle white rats were turned into attackers with the hypothalamus operation. They would lunge at anyone who opened their cage (as opposed to normal rats which are generally more timid), and if another rat was placed in the operated rat's cage, it would attack until the animal submitted. Two operated rats in the same cage would fight to the death. Another striking characteristic of these attack rats was their serum cholesterol level—it was severely elevated. Since one of the unequivocal laboratory techniques for inducing chronic coronary artery disease in animal models is to elevate serum cholesterol level, Drs. Friedman and Rosenman felt that they had simulated in animals the causal chain of aggressive, competitive personality leading to elevated cholesterol level which in turn led to heart disease.

There are four major lines of evidence which the cardiologists felt supported their contention that the Type A personality pattern leads to coronary heart disease. First, a great majority of those already suffering from heart disease could be classified as Type A's. Second, seemingly healthy individuals at the beginning of a period of study who were classified as Type A's were the individuals most likely to develop heart disease. Third, the biochemical abnormalities which are characteristic of coronary heart disease patients were also found in Type A people. Fourth, by making gentle rats into hostile, competitive Type A animals, high cholesterol levels were induced which led to coronary artery disease.

The research of Dr. Meyer Friedman and Dr. Ray Rosenman is the most extensive and convincing evidence of the relationship between personality and longevity. The work of Dr. George Gallup with near-centenarians, along with the research of many others on characteristics of long-lived people, had identified in these individuals the type of behavior pattern called Type B by Friedman and Rosenman. Although the earlier work was far less systematic and less conclusive, the similarity between descriptions of Type B's and centenarians is remarkable. According to Gallup, very long-lived people are "not upset by little things. They are—and have been—complacent, serene, unruffled, and self-possessed. There are no psychosomatic ailments here. Along with their heredity, light eating habits, and physical activity, their tranquility is one of the secrets of their longevity. Little wonder that Ponce de Leon never found the Fountain of Youth; he could not find it because he was seeking it."[8] Striving, pushing, and competing are life-shortening. The following description will help you determine if such deadly personality patterns characterize you.

HOW TO IDENTIFY THE TYPE A AND TYPE B BEHAVIOR PATTERNS

An extensive description of the Type A person is presented in Drs. Friedman and Rosenman's book, *Type A Behavior and Your Heart*. Excerpts from that description are provided here, but for the reader who suspects that he or she is a Type A person, it is strongly recommended that you also read the cardiologists' book which includes several chapters describing how to decondition yourself from this killing personality configuration. Here is what Feldman and Rosenman say is characteristic of Type A Behavior.

You Possess Type A Behavior Pattern:

1. If you have (a) a habit of explosively accentuating various key words in your ordinary speech even when there is no real need for such accentuation, and (b) a tendency to utter the last few words of your sentences far more rapidly than the opening words. The vocal explosiveness betrays the excess aggression or hostility you may be harboring. The hurrying of the ends of sentences mirrors your underlying impatience with spending even the time required for your own speech.

2. If you *always* move, walk, and eat rapidly.

3. If you feel (particularly if you openly exhibit to others) an impatience with the rate at which most events take place. You are suffering from this sort of impatience if you find it difficult to restrain yourself from hurrying the speech of others and resort to the device of saying very quickly over and over again, "Uh huh, uh huh," or "Yes, yes, yes, yes," to someone who is talking, unconsciously urging him to "get on with" or hasten his rate of speaking. You are also suffering from impatience if you attempt to finish the sentences of persons speaking to you before they can.

   Other signs of this sort of impatience: if you become *unduly* irritated or even enraged when a car ahead of you in your lane runs at a pace you consider too slow; if you find it anguishing to wait in a line or to wait your turn to be seated at a restaurant; if you find it intolerable to watch others perform tasks you know you can do faster; if you become impatient with yourself as you are obliged to perform repetitious duties (making out bank deposit slips, writing checks, washing and cleaning dishes, and so on), which are necessary but take you away from doing things you really have an interest in doing; if you find yourself hurrying your own reading or always attempting to obtain condensations or summaries of truly interesting and worthwhile literature.

4. If you indulge in *polyphasic* thought or performance, frequently striving to think of or do two or

more things simultaneously. For example, if while trying to listen to another person's speech you persist in continuing to think about an irrelevant subject, you are indulging in polyphasic thought. Similarly, if while golfing or fishing you continue to ponder your business or professional problems, or if while using an electric razor you attempt also to eat your breakfast or drive your car, or if while driving your car you attempt to dictate letters for your secretary, you are indulging in polyphasic performance. This is one of the commonest traits in the Type A man. Nor is he always satisfied with doing just two things at one time. We have known subjects who not only shaved and ate simultaneously, but also managed to read a business or professional journal at the same time.

5. If you find it *always* difficult to refrain from talking about or bringing the theme of any conversation around to those subjects which especially interest and intrigue you, and when unable to accomplish this maneuver, you pretend to listen but really remain preoccupied with your own thoughts.

6. If you almost always feel vaguely guilty when you relax and do absolutely nothing for several hours to several days.

7. If you no longer observe the more important or interesting or lovely objects that you encounter in your milieu. For example, if you enter a strange office, store, or home, and after leaving any of these places you cannot recall what was in them, you no longer are observing well—or for that matter enjoying life very much.

8. If you do not have any time to spare to become the things worth *being* because you are so preoccupied with getting the things worth *having*.

9. If you attempt to schedule more and more in less and less time, and in doing so make fewer and fewer allowances for unforeseen contingencies. A concomitant of this is a *chronic sense of time urgency*, one of the core components of Type A Behavior Pattern.

10. If, on meeting another severely afflicted Type A per-

son, instead of feeling compassion for his affliction you find yourself compelled to "challenge" him. This is a telltale trait because no one arouses the aggressive and/or hostile feelings of one Type A subject more quickly than another Type A subject.

11. If you resort to certain characteristic gestures or nervous tics. For example, if in conversation you frequently clench your fist, or bang your hand upon a table or pound one fist into the palm of your other hand in order to emphasize a conversational point, you are exhibiting Type A gestures. Similarly, if the corners of your mouth spasmodically, in tic-like fashion, jerk backward slightly exposing your teeth, or if you habitually clench your jaw, or even grind your teeth, you are subject to muscular phenomena suggesting the presence of a continuous *struggle,* which is, of course, the kernel of the Type A Behavior Pattern.

12. If you believe that whatever success you have enjoyed has been due in good part to your ability to get things done faster than your fellow men and if you are afraid to stop doing everything faster and faster.

13. If you find yourself increasingly and ineluctably committed to translating and evaluating not only your own but also the activities of others in terms of "numbers."[4]

Before you heave a sigh of relief after reading this description and say to yourself, "I'm not like that. I don't do all of those things," you should be aware that Friedman and Rosenman classify many people as Type A's who have a much lesser degree of these behavior patterns. The description above is of full-blown Type A behavior in all of its manifestations. It is only the rare individual who exhibits all of these behaviors. You should only feel safe if you are a true Type B. Unfortunately, few of us in the United States can meet the following criteria provided by Friedman and Rosenman as indicative of the Type B Behavior Pattern.

[4] From *Type A Behavior and Your Heart,* by Meyer Friedman and Ray H. Rosenman. © 1974 by Meyer Friedman. Reprinted by permission of Alfred A. Knopf, Inc.

You Possess Type B Behavior Pattern:

1. If you are completely free of *all* the habits and exhibit none of the traits we have listed that harass the severely afflicted Type A person.
2. If you never suffer from a sense of time urgency with its accompanying impatience.
3. If you harbor no free-floating hostility, and you feel no need to display or discuss either your achievements or accomplishments unless such exposure is demanded by the situation.
4. If, when you play, you do so to find fun and relaxation, not to exhibit your superiority at any cost.
5. If you can relax without guilt, just as you can work without agitation.[5]

Like the near-centenarians described by George Gallup, the Type B person is self-confident and seldom has his or her feelings hurt by opinions expressed by others. This individual has positive self-regard, along with a sense of humor which makes it easy to laugh at the inevitable mistakes he or she occasionally makes. They seek quality and experience rather than quantity and things. They take pleasure in simple beauty, noticing the smell of a flower or the green of the trees.

As in the case of the Type A Pattern, you may not exhibit all of the qualities of the full-blown Type B personality, but you can class yourself as a Type B if you are relatively free from all of the habits of a Type A person or if you exhibit only a few of them fairly rarely. For example, while you sometimes feel pressed for time, it is not a chronic condition and it occurs primarily on the job rather than at home or at play. Even on the job, to call yourself a Type B you should experience time pressure only infrequently. Type B's have other priorities in life so that the job never "gets to them" very much.

You may find it difficult to put yourself in the either/or categories of Type A or Type B, but Drs. Friedman and Rosenman believe that they can classify 90 percent of all people into one of the two categories. Before you make your final choice, consult your spouse or a close friend. Type A people seem to be particularly unaware of their rather unpleasant behavior pattern. If your spouse or friend gently suggests that you lean toward the Type A pattern, believe them, and count yourself among the individuals at high risk for a heart attack. Their gentle suggestion may put you on a path to change your habits, and that path may save your life.

CHANGING FROM TYPE A TO TYPE B

Usually in the case of Type A individuals it takes a brush with death to make them change their perspective, and even then it is extremely difficult to alter behavior patterns which have been sustained for years. Furthermore, many do not get the second chance because their first heart attack is often fatal.

One of the reasons that it is so difficult for Type A's to change is that they firmly believe that the rush they create for themselves is the thing that's getting them ahead. Their success in their occupation, they believe, has occurred because they accomplished things faster and got more jobs done than the peers with whom they compete. Little do they realize that their time pressured, competitive ways are probably holding them back and interfering with their true creative potential. Given time to analyze the junctures of their career, they might recognize that it was their talent or ideas rather than the number of reports they put out which got them ahead. Being so concerned with counting hours and numbers, however, prevents them from perceiving their actual worth, and they may actually hinder their career by continuing the mindless habits which they have come to believe are the reason for their success.

Drs. Friedman and Rosenman advocate a complete change of philosophy for Type A individuals. While these cardiologists recognize the tremendous difficulty involved in changing basic personality configurations, they believe that faced with almost certain death, many Type A's can and do change. Beginning with this premise that change can occur, certain guidelines are prescribed. One of the first things Friedman and Rosenman do is to get the Type A person to recognize that they have never failed because they did a job too well but too slowly. One accountant voiced this sentiment when he stated, "No matter how long I take to work on the books of a client, if I save him money, the client will return. On the other hand, whenever I rush and balance the books without time to find a savings, the client finds another accountant." Truly successful people recognize that quality at a slower pace is more valuable than quantity and speed. High quality work carried out at a slower rate seldom meets with disapproval, regardless of the occupation in which it is produced. However, work done too rapidly and poorly always brings complaints. Who would prefer paying a plumber slightly less for the time he spent on a job if he fixed the leak so poorly that it sprang open again in another month? There is no savings in such a situation.

Other suggestions provided by Friedman and Rosenman are to spend some time in self-appraisal to evaluate where you have been and where you are going. In this light the doctors also advise setting some long-term goals for your life and thinking about what will be important to you in your old age. Will you be able, like the near-centenarians described by George Gallup, to say that your life has been worthwhile and that you would do it the same way over again?

Attempting to regain your total personality, including those parts involving humor, appreciation for other people, and appreciation for life in general is another aspect of the physicians' prescription. They also feel that establishing some rituals and traditions in your life help to slow you down and to ground you in a more meaningful existence. Giving up many of the small, meaningless tasks you felt that only you could accomplish is another way to escape the time pressure, as is developing an attitude that unfinished jobs are not so undesirable. Deadlines apart from death are never final.

The main thrust of the guidelines, reengineering strategies, and drills provided by Friedman and Rosenman in their clinical practice and in *Type A Behavior and Your Heart* involve helping the Type A person to slow down, examine his or her life, and learn to enjoy it. In this regard, many of the exercises for relaxation presented in Chapter 13 can be helpful in changing the Type A Behavior Pattern, as can a daily fifteen-to-thirty-minute period of meditation. Yoga and Zen techniques and philosophy are particularly effective in combating patterns characteristic of Type A's, and this may explain in part why there is so much less cardiovascular disease in the East than in the West. Unfortunately, as countries such as Japan have become more industrialized and have adopted many of our Western ways, there has also been a startling increase in heart disease. That the centuries of Eastern tradition still have some protective effect is in evidence, however, in the fact that Japanese living in their own country have a lower incidence of coronary heart disease than Japanese who have migrated or who have been born in America.

At Colorado State University, Dr. Richard M. Suinn has developed what he calls the "Cardiac Stress Management Training Program" for individuals with the Type A behavior pattern. In this program patients learn to manage their anxiety when put in a high pressure situation, and they then learn to adopt alternative behaviors. The training lasts six weeks and uses techniques of muscle relaxation and visual imagery to help people cope. Learning to relax is the first step, and after the patient is relaxed he or she is asked to imagine a stressful scene. Relaxation is then fostered under the stressful stimulus, and the individual is trained to take control of the stressful event. The result of the sessions has been a change in behavior which was accompanied by a lowering of blood cholesterol level and blood pressure. Dr. Suinn commented that, "The Type A person, if he will make the effort, seems to be able to change his lethal lifestyle to a less risky one."[6]

The number one killing disease in the United States is associated with a number of poor health habits and with a personality pattern characteristic of the frontier spirit of aggressive competition and upward mobility. Excessive eating and smoking along with inactivity take a toll, but combined with feelings of time pressure, hostility, and competitiveness, these habits prove lethal to almost 800,000 Americans each year. Remarkably, all of these habits are things we can change, including the personality pattern which has been shown to be more deadly than most other leading causes of death combined.

OTHER DEADLY ASPECTS OF PERSONALITY

Adopting the Type A Behavior Pattern is probably one of the worst things you can do for your health and longevity, but there are other dangerous personality patterns which also result in premature death. A characteristic uniquely dangerous to younger individuals is risk-taking. Adopting daredevil traits and gaining attention by attempting crazy, dangerous feats, particularly in automobiles, are behavior patterns proving fatal to many Americans, especially young American males. The fourth greatest cause of death in our country is accidents, and they are the single greatest cause of death for all people between the ages of one and thirty-eight. Between the ages of five and twenty-four accidents claim more lives than do all other causes of death combined. That accidents are closely associated with daring and risk-taking is suggested by the fact that males, who learn to adopt such behavior patterns in far greater numbers than females, die three times as often from accidents as do females. Between the ages of 20–24, when young males are at their boldest and most daring, they die at a rate five times that of females. Men seem to become more careful in later adulthood, and the sex difference in accident rate almost disappears.

The number of deaths due to automobile accidents was almost as great as for all other accidents combined. It is clear that caution with automobiles lowers the risk. Using seat belts and driving at slower speeds prevent death. This was dramatically proved to the American public in 1974 when motor vehicle accident fatalities declined markedly as a result of the reduction in the mandatory speed limit to 55 miles per hour. That young males are the most likely to exceed speed limits and drive dangerously is evidenced by their much higher death rate in auto accidents and by the consequently higher insurance premiums they pay until the age 25 or 30.

Other needless deaths due to lack of caution occur as a result of falls, the second greatest accidental killer in our country. Carelessness resulting in fire leads to the third highest accidental killer, with drownings and poisonings following next in line. One of the reported personality changes which occurs with age is a shift to more cautious strategies. Many needless deaths would be avoided if this shift to caution emerged early in the life span.

Another element of danger in the risk-taking personality is the likelihood of involvement in crime and homicide. Homicide ranks thirteenth among the major causes of death in the United States, claiming over 16,000 lives per year. Only

France, among all the industrial nations of the world, has a higher homicide rate than the United States. Again, as in the case of accidents, the victims of homicide tend to be young. Homicide ranks second after accidents as the major killer of those between the ages of 15 and 24. Whether the high homicide rate in the United States is fostered by our frontier tradition, tensions experienced by the disadvantaged, and/or by excessive violence shown on television, we fail to eliminate the opportunity for aggressive individuals to kill one another by allowing easy access to handguns. Half of the homicide deaths occur from handguns, and guns are also responsible for another 13,000 deaths annually as a result of accidents and suicide.

Another deadly personality trait is depression, which frequently results in suicide. The eleventh major cause of death in the United States is suicide, accounting for over 22,000 deaths per year. Depression is a personality trait antithetical to the long-lived people studied by Gallup. However, while depression is related in a negative fashion to longevity, it seems to increase with age. There may be biological as well as social changes in old age precluding people to be more depressed. The old in contemporary society suffer from a number of physical, psychological, and social losses. Undoubtedly, these losses contribute to depression. That the major causes of depression are psychological and social rather than biological is evidenced by the fact that the suicide rate, the accompaniment of severe depression, does not rise dramatically with age for any group in the population except for white males. This phenomenon is shown dramatically in Figure 8. The causes for the high suicide rate in older white males are not clear, but it seems logical to associate it with the losses in physical and social prowess which are experienced by this group in the population which has known the most power and success up to the later years.

In addition to personality patterns involving risk-taking, aggression, and depression which can be shown to directly cause death, there are several personality traits which are correlated with earlier death which may or may not be causally related to it. A study of older people in Germany over a period of many years enabled researchers to predict survivors between the ages of 55 and 64 on the basis of certain personality characteristics. Among them was general dogmatism and rigidity. People who were more flexible in their attitudes and lives and less dogmatic about their beliefs survived longer.

Such a pattern again brings to mind characteristics common to most centenarians—the willingness to take life as it comes and adapt to changing circumstances. Dr. Robert Samp, a physician at the University of Wisconsin, emphasized this point after comparing the lifestyles of one thousand people over the age of 75 (including 129 centenarians) to the lifestyles of one thousand people who clinically were not expected to live much beyond 70. (The shorter-lived group ranged in age from 54 to 74 and included individuals who had heart disease, diabetes, and cancer.) Two key personality characteristics identified in the long-lived group were moderation and flexibility. Like the Type B individuals, the centenarians were not in a hurry. They had lived their 100 years in 100 years, while a lot of the members of the younger group

FIGURE 8 Suicide Rates, by Color, Sex, and Age, 1964.

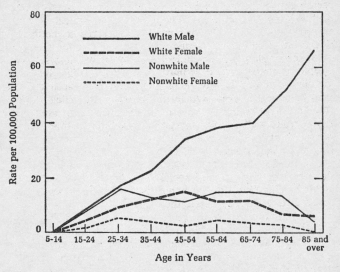

SOURCE: U.S. Department of Health, Education, and Welfare, "Suicide in the United States: 1950–1964," *Vital and Health Statistics* (data from the National Vital Statistics System), Series 20, No. 5. Washington, D.C.: U.S. Government Printing Office, 1967.

were burning out at 65 or 68. Their lack of rigid habits and their accommodation to change was another remarkable feature of the long-lived.

An extreme example of the ability to be flexible was presented by an old woman interviewed by Dr. Samp at the age of 101. This woman worked as a prostitute in the Western mining camps for over a decade in her youth, and then she married and had three children. Her husband and one of her children died, so to support her remaining brood, she ran a hotel and bar in Missouri and then opened a foster home for homeless children. When that home burned down, she moved with her widowed daughter to Colorado. The daughter had tuberculosis which the mother contracted. After spending two years in a sanitarium, at the age of 65 she married a fellow patient. They were both cured and bought a ranch in New Mexico. This remarkable woman ranched into her 80's, and at the time she was interviewed—over two decades later in Albuquerque—she claimed to Dr. Samp that her memory was "as clear as her record had become."[7] This ability to rebound from a life full of disasters and to retain a sense of humor and a clear mind attests to the flexibility characteristic of the long lived.

As a result of his extensive experience with longevous people, Dr. Samp has developed seven points which he feels can be fostered by parents in their children and in themselves. Adopting these personality characteristics early in life may help you to lead the kind of existence near the end of which you will find yourself a very interesting, content, long-lived person. The seven points are given in Table 5.

TABLE 5 Seven Common Denominators in the Very Old that You Can Develop in Yourself and Your Children

Oldsters	*You and your children*
1. Moderation	Moderate your "vices"—don't become an "addict" of anything.
2. Flexibility	Don't be rigid. Don't let your children "catch" your hangups—teach them to accept change.

3. Ability to "go one better"	Don't make life too easy for yourself or your children. Teach them not to give up, rather to push extra-hard at times.
4. Not preoccupied with health	Have a relaxed attitude toward health. Don't self-doctor or pill-pop.
5. Lack of concern with food and a "balanced" diet	Don't be a food faddist. Don't overemphasize quantity. Teach children to eat a wide variety of foods.
6. Activity and routine	Make activity part of every day. Teach your children to use their bodies regularly.
7. Concern for and contact with others	Keep in touch. Teach your children to care about people—to be outgoing[8]

Many of these points sound like the kind of advice which Drs. Friedman and Rosenman routinely give to their Type A patients and like the description of Dr. George Gallup in discussing the qualities of the long lived. The very similarities found by these experts, working in different specialities on different aspects of the concomitants of long life, suggest that there is a common thread of personality weaving itself through the fabric of a long life. Those who learn to have the most satisfying life—a life focused on happiness and on caring and interaction with others—are those who live the longest. What a pleasant conclusion to find after following several paths of long and rigorous scientific research endeavors. The best way to seek long life is to find happiness in the present.

CONCLUSION

15.

The Total Picture: Insuring a Long Future

&Ranging from heredity to personality, we have examined the relation of a wide variety of phenomena to longevity. The term *relation* must be emphasized, because in many cases the only data available are descriptions of characteristics of people who live the longest. We cannot say for sure that all of the qualities identified in longevous people *caused* them to live a long time. To be on the safe side, however, we may want to adopt many of these qualities for our own lives, knowing that future research efforts may demonstrate a causal relationship. In the following pages we will review all of the variables which appear to be related to longevity in an effort to summarize in a total package the things we can do to live a long time. We will also consider how some societies foster long life in an effort to determine what might be done on a national scale in the United States to make us the longest-lived country in the world.

WHAT YOU CAN DO, PERSONALLY

Through the longevity test you can determine how conducive your own personal heredity, health practices, education, occupation, and lifestyle are to longevity. Some of the factors which show the greatest relationships to longevity are things we cannot alter. Our sex, our race, and our parents' and grandparents' longevity are dramatically related to how long we live, and are things which we can hardly change, although in the case of sex, it has been shown that eunuchs live longer than intact men. Fortunately, there are ways we can compensate for these "givens" in our lives, apart from castration. In the case of sex differences in longevity, it appears that almost everything men can do to increase their longevity, women can do as well. Futrhermore, the benefits are often greater for women. Thus, at the present time, one of the most immutable inequalities in longevity is the sex difference. The more we improve the environment, the greater the life-expectancy gap between the sexes becomes. To women, this suggests the need to be most sensitive to the health and lifestyle changes they can make in their homes to teach their children and husbands habits conducive to long life. It also becomes apparent that men must discontinue several of the qualities characteristic of the "all-American" male—the aggressiveness, the push to get ahead as quickly as possible, the love for high-risk pastimes (particularly in automobiles) and the he-man diet loaded with calories, fats, and cholesterol.

Happily, one pastime to be encouraged in men and women is a rich and rewarding sexual life. Regular sexual activity, while it has not been shown to *cause* longer life in humans, is a habit characteristic in many longevous people. The zest for life, the stimulation, the exercise, and the close personal intimacy fostered by sexual activity may all contribute to its beneficial effects. This is one of the many cases in which quality of life enhances quantity. Who says we must give up everything we like to live a long time? Sex is a pleasure which should be indulged.

While the gap in life expectancy between the sexes continues to be maintained and even widened, life expectancy differences between the races are decreasing. This phenomenon demonstrates what a powerful effect the environment and alterations in the environment can have on longevity. Social and economic opportunity foster long life. Until that opportunity is equal for all Americans, we will have large racial differences in life expectancy which must stand as a national shame. That heredity could play a role in racial differences in longevity has been suggested and is reinforced by the fact that on average, Orientals live longer than Caucasians in the United States. However, this gap in life expectancy between Orientals and Caucasians is only about two years. When the black-white differences are reduced to that magnitude, perhaps then we can begin considering hereditary hypotheses. Blacks can play a personal role in this effort by doing such things as seeking medical attention to control hypertension, to which they seem particularly at risk. However, the total problem cannot be solved at a personal level, and society must be changed to be more conducive for opportunity and longevity among all segments of our population.

Heredity is something we cannot change, but we can be sensitized to our backgrounds to be alert to the kinds of life-shortening problems our parents and grandparents experienced, and we can take steps to avoid them. For example, knowing that coronary heart disease or arteriosclerosis runs in our family should be a particular warning signal for us to avoid the well-known risk factors. Maintaining a low cholesterol level by eating a low-fat, low-cholesterol diet, and by learning to avoid feelings of time pressure and hostile competition, keeping our blood pressure down by remaining slim and taking medication if necessary, exercising regularly, and not smoking are major things we can do to counteract a predisposition to heart disease. While a genetic component appears to exist in heart disease, many experts agree that it can be minimized if we would just stop killing ourselves with our habits. Smoking is about the craziest habit we can have from the perspective of longevity, particularly if a close relative has died of cancer. Low-fat diets also protect against a hereditary predisposition to cancer, as does the avoidance of pollutants in the environment. Particularly important in cancer is early detection. Thus, it is essential to have a physical examination every year and to be particularly careful to have genital areas examined annually, as these parts of the body are among the most vulnerable to cancer in both men and women.

In general, good health habits are essential to longevity. Diet is a major way in which we can intervene for long life. As Americans, we simply eat too much. One of the key words coming up again and again in discussions of longevity and in description of people who have lived to be 100 is *moderation.* Moderation in diet, in alcohol consumption, in exercise, in attitudes, in life changes, and in personality are conducive to living a long time. We simply must reduce the number of calories we eat to increase our life expectancy. In addition to eating less, we need to be more selective about what we eat. Eliminating high-fat, high cholesterol foods such as eggs, fatty beef, and fat-rich dairy products is as important as avoiding excess sugar. Preparation of food is important as well. Frying is not healthful, while broiling, boiling, poaching, baking, roasting, and barbecuing are. In addition, we need a well-balanced diet—with not a lot of any one kind of food (unless, of course, your physician is treating you for a special health condition).

Not enough can be said about the hazards of smoking. There is absolutely nothing healthful about smoking. There are so many other habits which you can develop to relax, that there is simply no excuse not to quit. Continuing to smoke is admitting to your family, your friends, and to yourself that you don't mind polluting their environment as well as your own, and you really don't love life enough to want to live as long as you can. Don't fool yourself that those extra years late in life won't matter. Most old people remark on how quickly life passes. Cutting it short is something you will live only long enough to regret.

Alcohol is a mixed blessing to which moderation is again the key. Its benefits to the circulation are so generally approved that it is often prescribed by physicians, particularly in old age. A glass or two of wine is touted for its effects as a relaxant, and as an aid to the digestive system. As a sleeping potent, it does wonders. How unfortunate, however, that such a substance can also be the source of more tragedy than any other drug. Excessive use of alcohol is one of the most life-shortening habits you can develop. So if you cannot drink moderately, then don't drink, and if you're a moderate drinker, be sure to maintain the moderation. For those who abstain—examine the evidence and make your choice. Just be tolerant, flexible, and relaxed about your views—that, too, is related to long life.

Exercise is another one of those habits which is related to life expectancy, but there are two important features to exercising for longevity. First, the activity must be regular—at least three and preferably four or five times a week. Second, moderation is important. Pushing yourself to the point of exhaustion where you overstress your body will not maximize your potential for long life. The number of joggers and even professional athletes who have died suddenly at a peak of exhaustion serves as a warning of the dangers of over-exertion. Make exercising into a pleasant part of your day, rather than a grueling endurance contest in which you punish yourself. Finding a partner or a group to share the activity will make it more enjoyable and perhaps more regular as you get some extra encouragement not to skip it "just this once." The type of exercise which involves your whole body is best, such as bicycling, jogging, swimming, brisk walking, skating, or dancing. The main point is to move, to increase your circulation, breathing, and muscle activity. Don't drive when you can walk, and try to be active on your job too. Saving labor has been seen as a boon in our society—but in terms of longevity, it has been a bust.

Sleeping too much is another way to be inactive, and too much sleep is correlated with a shorter life. The body needs to relax and refresh itself, and for most people this process takes six to eight hours per night. If life is so uninteresting that you prefer to spend almost half of it sleeping, or if you are so stressed that you cannot get more than five hours sleep per night, chances are you have some kind of problem. Evaluate and correct it yourself, or get professional help until your sleeping pattern returns to normal.

While it is easy to see specific ways in which we can change our health habits to enjoy longer life, our social status, determined by education, occupation, and income, may be more difficult to modify. Education has a direct bearing on our occupation, which in turn determines our income. Since the occupation and income of our parents affects our level of education, these three phenomena are not totally under our control, nor are they easily changed. Nevertheless, the higher the social status—that is, the higher the level of education, the category of occupation, and the income—the longer the life. Not only is it important to get as much education as possible, it is important to continue to learn and seek new educational experiences to improve the quality of life. Choosing an occupation which is suited to your interests and abilities is another way to maximize the positive manner in which occupation can affect your life. Finding a job in which you can succeed will affect your happiness and will reduce the stress you feel at work. Working in a stimulating, harmonious environment can have a positive effect on your health and life expectancy.

Occupational hazards which take such a great, and potentially avoidable toll in the occupational categories of skilled and unskilled laborers are often beyond the capabilities of the individual to change. One of the ways our society can foster long life is to stop tolerating the over 14,000 deaths which occur each year as a result of industrial accidents. Another way, mentioned previously, is to make opportunity more equally available for all. The life-shortening effects of poverty and low socioeconomic status are dramatic and need to be eradicated.

While research on longevity has demonstrated that there is no use in moving to the mountains or in seeking some perfect climate or geographical area that will extend your life, it has been shown that it is safer to live in the country than in the city. Those residing in rural areas live an average of two years longer than those inhabiting the city, and given all of the hazards more prevalent in cities, it is surprising that life expectancy differences between these two settings are not greater.

In addition to being a less dangerous environment, rural areas have other life-lengthening advantages. Occupations in the country tend to involve more activity, and farming is one of the healthiest occupations you can have. Access to fresh food, particularly fresh vegetables, is easier in the country, and the diets of rural dwellers may be healthier. The pace of life is also slower in the country, and close personal ties may be valued and stressed more. All of these factors make the country an easier and healthier place to live. If many of us cannot break our ties to the cities and move away, at least we can take a lesson from rural-urban differences affecting longevity and try to control our physical environment in such a way as to lessen the stress.

Stress results from a wide range of stimuli which can be physical, social, or psychological. Along with the environmental stressors such as noise, pollution, and crowding, excessive change has been identified as a factor harmful to health. Too many changes at one time—even ones that are positive—tax the adaptive capacities of an individual and make him or her vulnerable to a change in health. This suggests that we must attempt to regulate the number of changes occurring in our lives in a given year, and make decisions about changes with attention to what other circumstances will be happening in our lives at the time. As in the case of alcohol, exercise, and so many things in life, moderation in change is beneficial and leads to an interesting, stimulating life. Excessive change may land you in a hospital—or a grave.

Another form of stress in adulthood is living without close personal relationships. We have evolved as social beings, and social interaction appears to be essential for our health. It seems a bit odd in a book on longevity to advocate marriage, but the studies show that people who live intimately in stable relationships with members of the opposite sex live longer. But close personal relationships of all kinds are important. Most centenarians say that they love people, and they develop close personal ties to others. Having a close confidant increases life satisfaction in old age, and close friends and relatives are most important in cushioning against overwhelming sorrow and depression in times of personal crisis. Thus, the advice to cultivate close friendships and to find a partner with whom you can be happy for life is based on evidence gathered world-wide that humans survive best in the presence of close, loving others.

In addition to developing close personal ties to cope with the changes and stresses of life, several other strategies have proven successful. It is very important to be able to control the things which cause stress, even if this merely involves controlling the time at which you are exposed to the stressor. Taking a positive attitude toward the stressor is another way to control it, as is preparing yourself for exposure to it. This has been shown in the case of a stressful move for patients in nursing homes. If they know about the move, are helped to prepare for it, and are allowed to feel that they are participants in the process, the move will be far less stressful, and their chances of survival are greater.

Another very adaptive response to stress is to relax. If you can short-circuit the fast-beating heart, the sweaty palms, the faster breathing, and stomach butterflies which are some of our typical responses to stress by relaxing your muscles and your mind, you will remain in better health. While it is not an easy task to unlearn these innate, automatic responses to aversive situations, it is by no means impossible. Relaxation exercises and meditation are a way to do this. Even taking a few deep breaths or a brisk walk helps. Another aid is to change your perspective so that very few situations can make you upset.

People who have gotten so involved in the struggle for success that they have forgotten to enjoy life are not uncommon in the United States, for our system appears to nurture such behavior. This is one of the reasons that heart disease kills more of us than any other cause. Unfortunately, the people who are in the gravest danger are the least sensitive to their problem, and therefore are usually not motivated to change. Often, only a near-fatal heart attack can stop them long enough to re-evaluate their life and decide to work on changing their way of life. Many do not get this second chance.

Most of us know someone who has slowed down and learned to appreciate life and the people surrounding them as a result of a serious illness. Had this occurred years before the illness it would have been far more desirable, and it might even have prevented the illness. The heart attack victim's earlier misfortune and positive change can serve as a model for our own behavior and lead us to value personal happiness and deep interpersonal relationships over material success. When we adopt these values, material success seldom declines.

Another personality trait which kills a great number of American men, particularly young men, is the love of danger and of taking risks. Fifteen- to twenty-year-old men kill themselves behind the wheels of automobiles at an incredible rate. They also take risks which involve them in a greater number of other types of accidents *and* homicide. Modifying a risk-taking personality is not enough. We must also avoid carelessness.

Depression is another aspect of personality related to a shorter life. Suicide is frequently the direct result of depression, and older white men are particularly prone to this senseless end. One of the best counter-measures against depression is the development of close personal ties. Friends and relatives can play a critical role in times of trouble in helping the depressed individual to deal rationally with his or her life, and if they feel unable to perform this role alone, they should seek professional help.

The flexible, adaptive nature of centenarians is a characteristic noted by everyone who has studied their habits. Personality studies have also shown that people who are rigid and dogmatic tend to die younger than their more flexible contemporaries. Tension, anger, and hostility express themselves in the body in many negative ways, such as constriction of the arteries and hypertension, excessive flow of acid in the stomach, and excessive muscle constriction. Such bodily states, when maintained for long periods of time, result in headaches, ulcers, heart attacks, and strokes. Thus, if you find yourself getting too set in your ways, you may want to reevaluate your position. While too much change is also stressful, when you get to the point where you cannot tolerate changes in your life or differences in other people, you are losing your adaptability and as a result harming your health. This is another case where moderation is extremely important. Neither excessive change nor rigid stability is conducive to long life. We need to change and maintain our unique identity at the same time. Those of us who achieve this balance are the ones who live longest.

Societies Which Foster Long Life

There are a number of things which we can do personally to affect how long we live. At the same time, the society into which we are born places certain constraints within which we must operate. We are fortunate to be living in the United States at a time when the life expectancy is rising by a few months each year, placing it at an all-time high in 1976 for newborn males at 68.9 and for newborn females at 76.7. This average life expectancy of 72.8 is almost two years greater than the 70.9 year life expectancy in 1970 and is close to five years greater than life expectancy in 1949. If we look back to the turn of the century, we have added 25.5 years to the average person's life. This is the difference between dying before fifty, when the family is not even raised and out of the household, and living until grandchildren and possibly even great-grandchildren are born. It is the difference between having time for yourself after working and raising a family, and dying before any of your tasks are completed.

Although we are fortunate to live as long as we do today, we still have not responded well enough as a society to alleviate the things which are killing us before our program for life has run out. We are still almost thirty years short of 100, which is not even our full life-span potential. There are some places in the world where people live unusually long but which do not even have the public health advantages available in this country. Perhaps by examining the way of life in these societies we will be able to better understand what changes are necessary to foster longer life in the United States.

Of the three places in the world where extremely high concentrations of very long-lived people have been found, two of them—the Andean village of Vilcabanba in Ecuador, and the land of Hunza in Kashmir, Pakistan—are believed to be comprised of populations in which genetic selection is the major factor in the extreme longevity of the people. This is less true in Abkhasia in the U.S.S.R. because the region is not as isolated. Nevertheless, almost all of the very long-lived people, even in Abkhasia, had at least one long-lived parent or close relative. Low food intake and emphasis on activity and physical work throughout life are common to all three societies. Another aspect found in all of them is the tranquility of life, the lack of stress, and the regularity of their daily existence. There are no jarring transitions from one status to the next. Adolescence and old age do not find people changing roles dramatically, for they begin working in childhood and continue until they die. Retirement is not a part of life. Everyone has a place and a task.

Tradition has an important role in Abkhasia, and the old are the keepers of tradition. Their resources are highly valued and they are given high social status. Everyone respects the very old and plans and hopes to live that long. There is little loss in old age; rather there is gain: gain of prestige and influence.

Family ties and interpersonal relations are highly valued in this longevous society. Living together throughout their lives in small communities, the people develop a familiarity with one-another which few of us experience in our ever-mobile society. They avoid the stress of separation from loved ones and close friends by remaining in the towns where they were born.

There are some dramatic differences between life in the simple societies of Abkhasia, Hunza, and Vilcabanba and the complex industrial society in which we live, and there is no way we can ever change our society to approximate the tranquil, pastoral existence of these people. As a consequence, many more of us will die of stress-related diseases. This does not mean that there are no lessons we can learn from such societies. These groups and other facts we know about long life indicate alternatives we can institute to foster longevity in the United States.

SOCIETY'S ROLE IN LONG LIFE

As mentioned previously, efforts have continually been made in this country to improve the quality of life and health for the people. Those of us alive in this century are receiving the greatest benefit from this effort. However, we have not done all that is possible to insure the longest life to everyone. The following recommendations, based on research on longevity, are ways we could make life expectancy in the United States even greater.

Narrow the Gap Between the Poor and the Middle and Upper Income Groups

Large differences in life expectancy occur as a result of differences in education, occupation, and income. A major reason that poverty persists is because it creates a vicious cycle of lack of opportunity for the children of the poor. These children fail to get adequate education which prevents them from acquiring anything but low-paying and frequently dangerous jobs. Psychologists have documented the damage done to mental development by inadequate nutrition and stimulation which are characteristic of the infancy and early childhood of poor children. They begin school behind middle-class children, and they never catch up. They are far more likely to drop out of school at an early age, and by the time they are 12 to 14 their life pattern, including the probability of a short life span, is almost inevitably fixed.

Preschool intervention programs aimed at teaching parents how to facilitate mental growth in their children, and aimed also at stimulating the minds of the children themselves, have been shown to raise the performance of poor children to that comparable to their more fortunate peers. Such programs, along with pre- and post-natal nutrition programs, give at least some opportunity to those born in poverty to escape their life-shortening position. Nor should we give up on older generations of poor who have already suffered many of the set-backs associated with premature death. Programs insuring their health and income maintenance must continue, along with the creation of more jobs, adequate housing, and neighborhoods safe from crime.

That blacks and other minority group members constitute the greatest proportion of people in the poverty category is further evidence that poverty shortens life expectancy, because blacks live on the average of five years less than whites. The fact that unequal opportunity, determined by something as random as skin color, can cut years off of life in the United States is antithetical to the principles on which our society is based. While some say that we can no longer afford social programs to spread opportunity more equally among people, in terms of the cost in suffering and years of human life we cannot afford not to expand such programs. In this manner we can become more like the Netherlands and the Scandinavian countries in which life expectancy shows almost no variance as a function of social class. Those countries also have the highest average life expectancy in the world.

Reduce the Infant Mortality Rate

Coupled with the lack of opportunity at all ages for some population groups in the United States is the disproportionately high infant mortality rate suffered in lower socioeconomic groups. Such inequities make the infant mortality rate in the United States 20th in the world. Although the infant mortality rate has dropped from 55.7 (that is, 55.7 deaths among babies under one year of age for every 1,000 born) in 1935 to 16.1 in 1975, there is still much we can do to eliminate death among babies. That this is possible has been demonstrated in Sweden where in 1970 the infant mortality rate was 11.0. Making high-quality prenatal care available to every mother in the United States would help to make this possible, and special attention must continue to be focused on young (under 20), poor and/or black mothers among whom the infant mortality rate is greatest. Lack of education or money causes these women to get little or no prenatal or postnatal care, and the infant mortality rates among these groups give evidence to the harm caused by this lack. The infant mortality rate among American nonwhites is 31.0, which is almost twice the infant mortality rate for whites. From the time they are conceived, members of certain sub-groups in our population are disadvantaged. There is little that these individuals can do personally to extend their life expectancy. As a society, we must take action for them.

Lower Industrial Accident Rates

While modern industry has given Americans the highest standard of living in the world, it continues to take a toll in lives which could and must be avoided. In 1972, there were 14,200 accidental deaths on the job, and 2,300,000 workers suffered disabling injuries at work. This toll is the visible evidence of our scandalous record of industrial safety. The impossible-to-measure number of deaths resulting from industrial pollutants and industrial poisoning affects tens of thousands more. Stricter safety laws legislated at state and federal levels are one way to reduce this hazard. Regulations should extend not only to dangerous equipment, but also to poisons, pollutants, and noise. In addition to looking to the government to force us to manufacture more safely, the impetus should also come from the private sector—from concerned consumer groups and environmentalists, and from workers, plant managers, and corporation heads.

Reduction of Automobile Accidents

The envirionmental crisis which forced the lowering of the maximum speed limit proved to us that we have it in our power to reduce fatalities on the road, yet as we relax those standards and the enforcement of them, the automobile fatality rate is increasing again. Since its invention, the automobile has killed a total over two million Americans—more than in all of this nation's wars. Auto deaths could be reduced by a third if we would all wear our seat belts at all times. Since even at the risk of serious injury and death the great majority of us fail to take such precautions, it is time to install protective inflatable devices and automatic seat belts which we cannot fail to use. The licensing laws could also be made stricter in those states and localities which in some cases allow children of 14, mental defectives, drug addicts, and semi-blind individuals to drive. Periodic re-licensing would also reduce the number of incompetent drivers on the road, as would more severe penalties such as revocation of the driving license for individuals, particularly drunks, who demonstrate that they are a life-threatening menace on the road. In Sweden it is routine for police to stop drivers and check the alcohol content of their blood. If they have had more than one drink or two beers (resulting in more than an .05 percent blood alcohol content level), they are sentenced to up to six months in jail. This procedure has made it a social norm in Sweden that the driving member of a group does not drink, and a lower rate of auto fatalities is the result. State-enforced automobile safety checks required at regular intervals would also prevent more accidents resulting from defective machinery.

In addition to the direct manner in which we outright kill in auto accidents, we shorten our lives through the inactivity brought about by our habit of driving everywhere. Ours is the automobile lifestyle. We seldom walk when we can ride. Conditioning ourselves to leave the car in the garage and walk to our destination or to public transportation is one easy way to insure daily exercise, and it also cuts down on air pollution. One of the fortunate consequences of our rapidly declining environmental resources may be to prevent us from using our cars so much. With the price of gasoline at $1.50 a gallon, the payoff of walking will become more evident.

Improvement of the Purity of Air, Water and Food

The second leading cause of death in our country, cancer, may be almost totally caused by environmental pollutants. Even mental health problems, including hyperactivity in children and premature senility in old people, have recently been associated with additives in food and even in food packaging. This problem has received national attention and caused some, such as Dr. Michael Lesser of the University of California at Berkeley, to call for a Bill of Rights for Clean Air, Water, and Pure Food. We are simply too casual as individuals about what we put into our bodies and as a society about what we will tolerate in our environment. Noise, crowding, and pollution stress our lives, yet we prefer to try to adapt and die at a younger age. Indeed, the Food and Drug Administration policies on Laetrile and saccharine have stirred up such a public outcry that many are becoming critical of the government's role in legislating public health standards. It appears that we prefer the freedom to choose to die from a cancer cure which has been proven ineffective or to risk developing cancer by ingesting a probable carcinogen to having the government make the choice for us. Such a mood seems odd at a time when health food and exercise are at an all-time high in terms of the number of enthusiasts they are attracting. Unfortunately, freedom of choice is not always conducive to longevity. Countless articles and programs are in evidence which implore us to stop killing ourselves, yet many of us have not learned to love life enough to make its preservation a high priority. We fail to think of our later years. This may change, however, as we age as a nation, and old people are in greater evidence. Their presence may help us to become more conscious about preserving our own lives.

Another recent environmental policy is the emphasis to switch to coal as a primary source of energy, even if it means relaxing envirionmental standards. Since coal was first mined in England early in the 14th century, people have been aware of its hazards. Surely we should not be willing to sacrifice some of our gains in life expectancy for cheaper energy. While the options available in this matter may be limited, the pendulum of societal attitudes should not be allowed to swing back to the point where we no longer concern ourselves with the purity of the environment. Otherwise we will be paying a price with our lives.

Reduction of the Homicide Rate

The most efficient way to cut short a life is murder, and we Americans are overly proficient in this life-shortening technique. Our homicide rate is the second highest in the world, and we lose many members of our population, particularly our youth, to this cause of death. One way to reduce its toll would be to more strictly regulate the sale and ownership of guns. Another way, one in which we are presently making some progress, is to reduce the amount of violence shown on television and in films.

It has been estimated that if accidents and homicide were cut in half in the United States, almost one year would be added to the average life expectancy. We currently know more about how to accomplish such reductions than we do about curing cancer and heart disease. We should be willing to act on this knowledge.

Abolishment of Retirement

One of the primary characteristics of Abkhasian society credited with the prolongation of life is the role and status given to old people and the stability of their work role over the life span. The abrupt change in status experienced as a result of retirement is stressful to most individuals at a time in their lives when it is not as easy to deal with stress. While we cannot conclusively say that retirement causes death, we do know that life and health are improved in individuals who feel needed, who have adequate financial resources, and who have high social status. The loss of a job resulting from mandatory retirement at the age of 65 deprives individuals of these life-sustaining variables. Those who continue to work after the age of 65 have fewer depressive episodes than those who retire or who are unemployed. Many continue to work if they can, regardless of how it affects their income. They appear to have a desire to remain useful or creative rather than to disengage. High morale, adjustment, and a sense of belonging, all characteristics of centenarians, are found more often among those not forced to retire. We may be shortening life expectancy by imposing mandatory retirement, and we are clearly writing off an important national resource—the wisdom accumulated through years of experience.

Congress and the President seem determined to end mandatory retirement on the basis of age in the next several years, and there is much public support for this legislation. Rather than see it as a threat to jobs for the young, we should see it as an opportunity for people of all ages to shift to a lifestyle in which time spent in work and leisure are more equally spread. Rather than an abrupt change from full-time employment to retirement, old people should enjoy a gradual shift from more hours working to more hours free. If work and leisure were more integrated at all points of the life span, this transition would be even easier. Four-day work weeks and periodic sabbaticals for everyone would allow fuller employment and greater enjoyment of life. Such scheduling might help us to be less oriented to the act of producing and to the material goods produced, and more oriented to the quality of our lives. We would have more time for recreation and education, and more time to spend with family and friends. Such changes in the quality of life might have a dramatic impact on the quantity.

Elimination of "Agism"

The aged suffer from a tremendous amount of discrimination. It has been suggested that we should re-educate the whole population of young and middle-aged people to eradicate their prejudice against old people. Such attitudes are damaging to the individuals who are old, and they set up a situation which becomes a self-fulling prophecy. If you anticipate old age to be a time of decline, it will be. But if you meet it with the attitude that it is as good a time in life as any other, it will be that instead.

In his recently published book, *A Good Age,* Alex Comfort points out that "agism" is society's most stupid bias. The elderly are the only outcast group that everyone eventually will join. The argument presented by Dr. Comfort is that the chief disability in old age is agism itself. In societies such as in Abkhasia, where old age enjoys a particularly high status, people survive longer. In our society death occurs because there is no longer a desire to live. Many old people may die too soon because of agism. Most of the handicaps of being old in the United States are social, conventional, and imaginary, according to Dr. Comfort. As a biologist he is willing to admit that the physical changes which occur with age are trifling in comparison to the social consequences of being old. Most of the reputed declines of old age are a myth. One of the greatest of these is the myth of senility. Loss of mental facilities is hardly an inevitable consequence of old age, and it is extremely rare. Only one percent of the elderly can expect to become demented. Less than 5 percent of people over the age of 65 are institutionalized at any one time, and only about 15 percent of old people will ever be in an institution.

Alex Comfort believes that the elderly are patronized, overmedicated, and arbitrarily exluded from any significant social roles, and he encourages them to do something about it. Among his tips involving consciousness raising is to take no guff about age. He insists that any titles such as "Pop" or "Granny" must be eliminated, and their users punished. To the rigid attitudes of physicians, Dr. Comfort states that old people must be firm, particularly if any problem is brushed off as "simply due to age." He tells the story of the old man of 104 who complained of a stiff knee and was told that he couldn't expect to be agile at his age. To this the man responded that he'd had the other knee for 104 years too, and it wasn't stiff!

While some of these tactics seem antithetical to the typical centenarian, traits of moderation and of taking life as it comes, the humor and self-respect advocated by Dr. Comfort is typical of the long lived. We certainly would not want to turn people at the age of 65 into a generation of angry Type A's. However, it is a tragedy to see so many of our older people waste away in depression. Such is not the inevitable end of life, as studies of centenarians and of long-lived peoples throughout the world have proved.

Invest in More Research on Longevity and Aging

It is only in the last century, when science has finally been allowed to flourish, that the greatest gains in human longevity in the course of history have occurred. All but a few of us owe most of the years of our survival to medical break-throughs. There is no doubt that future advances can be made to extend life expectancy and to eliminate chronic diseases such as heart disease and cancer. What is in doubt is the pace at which these advances will occur. Depending on the amount of resources we are willing to divert to research on aging, those of us alive today will survive a shorter or longer period.

In addition to research on the biological, psychological, social, and environmental causes of chronic diseases, we need to know a great deal more about the causes of differences in longevity resulting from sex, race, social class, and marital status. Why are there such great gaps in life expectancy between these groups, and how can the gaps be narrowed? A national policy aimed toward equalizing life expectancy for every individual born in the United States should be instituted, and to implement such a policy we must have more facts. How can we intervene to make men live as long as women? There are a few suggestive answers, but we really have little to go on. The large life expectancy differences as a function of marital status is a phenomenon familiar to few scientists, and almost no research has been undertaken to determine its cause.

In response to the growing numbers of old people in our society, Congress created the National Institute of Aging in 1974 to focus on some of these basic research issues and to stimulate new research in gerontology. The amount of resources diverted to this institute in the last several years is relatively small, considering the magnitude of the problem of aging. This Institute is one of three relatively new agencies created to attack the problems of aging. The others are the Administration on Aging, which supports direct service programs to the elderly along with programs of applied research and training, and the Center for the Study of Aging and Human Development, which supports research on mental health and aging. The programs supported by these agencies have the potential to accelerate the pace at which we expand knowledge about longevity and aging. The outcome of such knowledge will be the development of means to extend life expectancy and, ultimately, life span. The greater our investment in this research, the longer our lives will extend into the twentieth and twenty-first centuries.

16.

Epilogue: Can We Live to Be 300?

&The purpose of this book has been to identify factors related to a full and long life. We have talked of the human life span as fixed and final at around 120 years, and we have discussed phenomena which improve or hinder our chances of reaching that upper limit. However, gerontology, the scientific study of aging, has more to its goal than the mere elimination of diseases and social and environmental hazards which prevent us from living to be 120. A significant portion of the research in gerontology is aimed at identifying the basic nature of the aging process and at discovering a means to extend the human life span. Furthermore, more than a few gerontologists believe that we are not far off from doing just that. The frontier of gerontological research may be pushing very near to the causes of biological aging, and once we know the causes, prevention of aging will not be far off.

To many who are unaware of the extensive amount of research being carried out on the biology of aging, the suggestion that we are nearing the discovery of the ultimate causes of death comes as a shock. The prospect that we may be able to extend the human life span to 300 or 1,000 or more years appears even more bizarre. But then, who would have imagined that we'd fly around the world in jumbo jets, or that we'd land on the moon, or that we'd find a cure for polio? Arthur C. Clarke, the science fiction writer, commented that whenever an expert insists that a problem is impossible to solve, he is certainly premature and almost certainly mistaken. Thus, although the skeptical question whether we will ever be able to unlock the complexities of the human body to the point where we can reprogram it, many scientists agree that it is just a matter of time.

How much time will it take? Will any of us alive today be around to see or derive the benefits of the extension of the life span? It is impossible to set up a precise timetable for scientific advancement in gerontology, but some gerontologists working on the causes of aging have made predictions. Dr. Donner Denckla, working at The Roche Institute of Molecular Biology in New Jersey, believes that he is on the track of discovering why we die, and he has estimated the various steps he will have to go through before he has a drug on the market to prolong life. He thinks it will take 40 years! Furthermore, Dr. Denckla believes that with stepped-up funding and expanded facilities, he might be able to get the job done in half that time. This means that most people alive today could benefit and extend their life span. While Dr. Denckla might be called an *avant garde* gerontologist, he is respected in the field as a serious scientist. His predictions will clearly be tested in laboratories across the country and throughout the world.

A famous Russian gerontologist, Dr. Zhores A. Medvedev predicts that by the middle of the 21st century we will live to 150–160 years. Medvedev believes that a long life will make us more humanitarian. In answer to the question, "Why extend the life span?" Medvedev answers: "We are merely attempting to make our life better because it is too short. If it were longer, people might savor it in less haste and perhaps with more altruism. This is why I believe that the work of prolonging human life is not an irresponsible social project."[1]

After interviewing gerontologists throughout the country, Albert Rosenfeld, science editor of *Saturday Review*, recently wrote a book about extending the life span called *Prolongevity*. From his experience in the gerontological laboratories across the country, this leading scientific journalist concludes, "I will venture to predict that by the year 2025—if research proceeds at reasonable speed—most of the major mysteries of the aging process will have been solved, and the solutions adopted as part of conventional biomedical knowledge; and that some of the solutions will by then already have come into practical use to stave off the ravages of senescence."[2] The year 2020 has been named by some as the year of the gerontology boom because the large group of people born in the post-World War II baby boom will be 65 to 70 at that time. If Albert Rosenfeld is correct, this large group will be among the first to experience the real benefits of basic gerontological research.

Another group is also hoping to benefit from breakthroughs in gerontology, although many of these people will not live beyond the next twenty years. This group of people belong to the cryonics movement launched by Robert Ettinger when he published *The Prospect of Immortality*. Instead of burial or cremation, Ettinger proposed the freezing of dead bodies to preserve them until the day when medical science has advanced to a point where aging and death are eliminated. The prospects for success in such an endeavor are extremely remote, but Ettinger, a professor of physics, wins adherents to his movement by convincing them that the chances of returning to life are not zero. The only thing people in the cryonics movement have to lose is money. As of 1975, the initial cost of freezing was $15,000, and maintenance charges cost $1,800 per year. Cryonics societies, which exist in several parts of the United States, point out that a $50,000 life insurance policy would cover all costs. The official number of people who have carried out this plan, according to Albert Rosenfeld, is around 25, although he suggests that many more cryonic interments may have taken place secretly.

This group, seeking life even in death, has really no more unusual approach than many of the methods attempted throughout history. The famous scientist, patriot, statesman, and great American, Benjamin Franklin, predicted that some day the human life span would be 1,000 years, and for himself he mused:

> I wish it were possible, from this instance, to invent a method of embalming drowned persons, in such a manner that they may be recalled to life at any

period, however distant, for having a very ardent desire to see and observe the state of America a hundred years hence, I should prefer to any ordinary death, the being immersed in a cask of Madeira wine, with a few friends, till that time, to be then recalled to life by the solar warmth of my dear country. But . . . in all probability we live in an age too early and too near the infancy of science to hope to see an art brought in our time to its perfection . . .

Franklin, one of the first great American scientists, envisioned an era which contemporary American gerontologists 200 years later are beginning to make a reality. While the frontier of gerontological research is in flux, more and more scientists are acknowledging the possibility that there is a program or "clock of aging" determining how long we live. Even more importantly, they are agreeing that this biological clock may be identifiable and reprogrammable. Some believe that the clock resides in the cells, others argue that it must lie in the brain, while still others are seeking the key in the genetic material, the DNA. None of these approaches may be wrong, as there may be several clocks intricately orchestrated by the genes. Tbe exciting fact is that so many scientists are ready to admit the real possibility of altering the program for life— not in the far distant future, but now.

Without doubt, the profound social consequences of such a discovery will create tremendous problems. Almost every aspect of human experience and expectation would be altered. Do we want such a change? Could we cope with it? Perhaps the best thing to do would be to look to the oldest and most longevous among us: those who already know the secrets to living a long life, those who have lived to be 100. Given what we have learned about these well-adjusted, adaptable people, we might suspect that they would react to the extension of the life span as they have reacted to life throughout their years. They would accept it, adapt to it, and learn to enjoy it.

Appendix

Bicentennial Charter for Older Americans

Two hundred years ago, a new nation was founded based on the self-evident truths that all men—and women are created equal and that they are endowed by their Creator with certain inalienable rights. A Constitution was set forth for governance of these new United States of America with the goal of forming a more perfect union, establishing justice, insuring domestic tranquillity, providing for the common defense, promoting the general welfare, and securing the blessings of liberty to ourselves and our posterity.

In the two hundredth year of this nation's existence, it is good and well that we call special attention to a group of citizens which literally did not exist at the time of our Revolution. The life expectancy at birth in 1776 was 32 years. In 1976, it is projected to be 71 years and we now have a virtual "generation" of older Americans whose roles, contributions, rights and responsibilities need to be given particular attention at this time in our history.

Americans of all ages have the ultimate responsibility to be or become self-reliant, to care for their families, to aid their neighbors and to plan prudently for their old age. Older persons have the responsibility to make available to the community the benefits of their experience and knowledge. Society—be it through the institutions of the public or the private sector—has the responsibility to assist citizens to be prepared for their later years as well as to assist directly so many of the very old who for one reason or another cannot cope with the burden of increasing physical, mental, social and environmental debilities.

There follow certain basic human rights for older Americans based on the "laws of nature and of nature's God" as set forth in the founding documents of this nation some two hundred years ago.

I   **The Right of Freedom, Independence and the Free Exercise of Individual Initiative.**

This should encompass not only opportunities and resources for personal planning and managing one's life style but support systems for maximum growth and contributions by older persons to their community.

II   **The Right to an Income in Retirement Which Would Provide an Adequate Standard of Living.**

Such income must be sufficiently adequate to assure maintenance of mental and physical activities which delay deterioration and maximize individual potential for self-help and support. This right should be assured regardless of employment capability.

III   **The Right to an Opportunity for Employment Free from Discriminatory Practices Because of Age.**

Such employment when desired should not exploit individuals because of age and should permit utilization of talents, skills and experience of older persons for the good of self and community. Compensation should be based on the prevailing wage scales of the community for comparable work.

IV   **The Right to an Opportunity to Participate in the Widest Range of Meaningful Civic, Educational, Recreational and Cultural Activities.**

The varying interests and needs of older Americans require programs and activities sensitive to their rich and diverse heritage. There should be opportunities for involvement with persons of all ages in programs which are affordable and accessible.

V   **The Right to Suitable Housing.**

The widest choices of living arrangements should be available, designed and located with reference to special needs at costs which older persons can afford.

VI   **The Right to the Best Level of Physical and Mental Health Services Needed.**

Such services should include the latest knowledge and techniques science can make available without regard to economic status.

VII   **The Right to Ready Access to Effective Social Services.**
These services should enhance independence and well-being, yet provide protection and care as needed.

VIII   **The Right to Appropriate Institutional Care When Required.**
Care should provide full restorative services in a safe environment. This care should also promote and protect the dignity and rights of the individual along with family and community ties.

IX   **The Right to a Life and Death With Dignity.**
Regardless of age, society must assure individual citizens of the protection of their constitutional rights and opportunities for self respect, respect and acceptance from others, a sense of enrichment and contribution, and freedom from dependency. Dignity in dying includes the right of the individual to permit or deny the use of extraordinary life support systems.

We pledge the resources of this nation to the ensuring of these rights for all older Americans regardless of race, color, creed, age, sex or national origin, with the caution that the complexities of our society be monitored to assure that the fulfillment of one right does not nullify the benefits received as the result of another entitlement. We further dedicate the technology and human skill of this nation so that later life will be marked in liberty with the realization of the pursuit of happiness.

TABLE 6   Cookbooks on Low-Fat and Low-Cholesterol Foods and Their Preparation

Belinkie, H.: *The Low-Fat Cookbook for Gourmets.* New York: D. McKay, 1964.

Bond, C., E. V. Dobbin, H. F. Gofman, H. C. Jones, and L. Lyon: *The Low-Fat Cholesterol Diet,* 2nd ed., New York: Doubleday, 1971.

Cavanna, E., and J. Welton: *Gourmet Cookery for a Low-Fat Diet.* Englewood Cliffs, N. J.: Prentice-Hall, 1961.

Rosenthal, S.: *Life High on Low-Fat.* Philadelphia: Lippincott, 1962.

Stead, E. A., and J. V. Warren: *Low-Fat Cookery,* 3rd ed., New York: McGraw-Hill, 1975.

TABLE 7 Approximate Cholesterol Content of Selected Foods

Item	Portion	Size, gm	Cholesterol per edible portion, mg
Beef, cooked, trimmed	4 oz.	113	102
Cooked, untrimmed	4 oz.	113	113
Brains, cooked, no fat added	3 oz.	85	2,674
Butter	1 pat	7	20
Cheese: cheddar and processed	1 oz.	28	45
Cottage, creamed	1 cup	225	23
Cream	1 oz.	28	36
Spreads and cheese foods	1 oz.	28	39
Chicken, turkey, cooked	4 oz.	113	85
Cream: light (20% fat)	1 tbsp.	15	11
Half and Half (12% fat)	1 tbsp.	15	6
Egg: whole	1 med.	50	235
White	1 med.	33	0
Yolk	1 med.	17	235
Fish, lean and medium fat, cooked	4 oz.	113	79
Very fat, cooked	4 oz.	113	90
Gefilte fish	3 oz.	85	54
Heart, cooked	3 oz.	85	119
Ham, cooked, trimmed	4 oz.	113	102
Cooked, untrimmed	4 oz.	113	113
Ice cream	1 scoop	71	43
Ice milk	1 scoop	71	4
Kidney, cooked, no fat added	3 oz.	85	298
Lamb, cooked, trimmed	4, oz.	113	102
Cooked, untrimmed	4 oz.	113	113
Lard and other animal fat	1 tbsp.	14	14–17
Liver, cooked, no fat added	3 oz.	85	213
Margarine, all vegetable fat	1 pat	7	0
Mayonnaise and mayonnaise-type salad dressing	1 tbsp.	14	8
Milk: fluid, whole	1 cup	244	27
Fluid, skim	1 cup	246	0
Pork, cooked, trimmed	4 oz.	113	102
Cooked, untrimmed	4 oz.	113	113
Shellfish: clams, crab, lobster, mussels, shrimp, cooked	4 oz.	113	170
Sweetbreads, cooked	3 oz.	85	249

Tongue, cooked fresh	3 oz.	85	119
Cooked smoked	3 oz.	85	179
Veal, cooked, trimmed	4 oz.	113	102
Cooked, untrimmed	4 oz.	113	113

NOTE: Cholesterol is not present in foods of plant origin such as fruits, vegetables, cereal grains, legumes, nuts or oils.

SOURCE: Latham, M. C., R. B. McBandy, M. B. McCann, and F. J. Stare: *Scope Manual on Nutrition*. Kalamazoo, Mich.: Upjohn Co., 1970. By permission of the Upjohn Co., Kalamazoo, Mich. 49001.

Bibliography

CHAPTER 1

Bell, A. G.: The Duration of Life and Conditions Associated with Longevity, a Study of the Hyde Genealogy. Washington, D.C.: Genealogical Record Office, 1918.

Friedman, M., and R. H. Rosenman: *Type A Behavior and Your Heart.* New York: Alfred A. Knopf, 1974.

Holmes, T. H., and R. H. Rahe: "The Social Readjustment Rating Scale," *Journal of Psychosomatic Research*, 1967, **11**, 213–218.

Kitagawa, E. M., and P. M. Hauser: *Differential Mortality in the United States: A Study in Socioeconomic Epidemiology.* Cambridge, Mass.: Harvard University Press, 1973.

Metropolitan Life Insurance Company: "Centenarians," *Statistical Bulletin*, 1971, **52**, 3–4.

Metropolitan Life Insurance Company: "Mortality Differentials Among Non-white Groups," *Statistical Bulletin*, 1974, **55**, 5–8.

Metropolitan Life Insurance Company: "Socioeconomic Mortality Differentials," *Statistical Bulletin*, 1975, **56**, 3–5.

Metropolitan Life Insurance Company: "Expectation of Life Among Nonwhites," Statistical Bulletin, 1977, **58**, 5–7.

Metropolitan Life Insurance Company: "Longevity in the United States at New High," *Statistical Bulletin*, 1977, **58**, 9–11.

Reinhold, R.: "New Population Trends Transforming U.S.," *The New York Times*, February 6, 1977.

U.S. Bureau of the Census: *Census of the Population, 1970. Vol I, Characteristics of the Population (Part I—U.S. Summary)*. Washington, D.C.: U.S. Government Printing Office.

U.S. Department of Health, Education, and Welfare: "Mortality Trends for Leading Causes of Death: United States 1950–1969," *Vital and Health Statistics*, Series 20, No. 6. Washington, D.C.: U.S. Government Printing Office, 1974.

CHAPTER 2

Burke, T.: "Romania's Remarkable Rejuvenator Gerovital H_3," *Town & Country*, January, 1973, 1–2, 10, 18–19.

Comfort, A.: *The Process of Ageing*. New York: New American Library, 1964.

Cutler, N. E., and R. A. Harootyan: "Demography of the Aged," in D. S. Woodruff and J. E. Birren (eds.), *Aging: Scientific Perspectives and Social Issues*. New York: Van Nostrand, 1975, pp. 31–69.

Dublin, L. I., A. J. Lotka, and M. Spiegelman: *Length of Life: A Study of the Life Table*. New York: Ronald Press, 1949.

Gruman, G. J.: "A History of Ideas About the Prolongation of Life: The Evolution of Prolongevity Hypothesis to 1800," *Transactions of the American Philosophical Society*, 1966.

Lynn, N.: "Rejuvenation Clinics," *Harper's Bazaar*, August, 1975, 18, 81.

Metropolitan Life Insurance Company: "International Trends in Longevity," *Statistical Bulletin*, 1974, 35, 9–11.

Spiegelman, M., and C. L. Erhardt: "Mortality and Longevity in the United States," in C. L. Erhardt and J. E. Berlin (eds.), *Mortality and Morbidity in the United States*, Cambridge, Mass.: Harvard University Press, 1974, pp. 1–20.

United Nations: *Demographic Yearbook: 1972*. New York: The United Nations, 1973.

U.S. Public Health Service, National Center for Health Statistics: *Monthly Vital Statistics Report* 22: 13. Washington, D.C.: U.S. Government Printing Office, 1974.

Weg, R. B.: "Changing Physiology of Aging: Normal and Pathological," in D. S. Woodruff and J. E. Birren (eds.), *Aging: Scientific Perspectives and Social Issues*. New York: Van Nostrand, 1975, pp. 229–256.

CHAPTER 3

Auerbach, S.: "Women Increase Age Gap," *Philadelphia Inquirer*, January 11, 1977.

Benet, S.: *Abkhasians: The Long-Living People of the Caucasus.* New York: Holt, Rinehart and Winston, 1974.

Butler, R.: "Sex After Sixty," in L. Brown and E. Ellis (eds.), *The Later Years.* Acton, Mass.: Publishing Sciences, 1975.

Comfort, A.: *The Process of Ageing.* New York: New American Library, 1964.

Cutler, N. E., and R. A. Harootyan: "Demography of the Aged," in D. S. Woodruff and J. E. Birren (eds.), *Aging: Scientific Perspectives and Social Issues.* New York: Van Nostrand, 1975, pp. 31–69.

Drori, D., and Y. Folman: "The Effect of Mating on the Longevity of Male Rats," *Experimental Gerontology,* 1969, **4,** 263–266.

Drori, D., and Y. Folman: "Environmental Effects on Longevity in the Male Rat: Exercise, Mating, Castration, and Restricted Feeding," *Experimental Gerontology,* 1976, **11,** 25–32.

Feinleib, M.: "Changes in Life Expectancy Since 1900," *Circulation,* 1975, **52,** 16–17.

Golde, P., and N. Kogan: "A Sentence Completion Procedure for Assessing Attitudes Toward Old People," *Journal of Gerontology,* 1959, **14,** 355–363.

Kinsey, A. C., W. B. Pomeroy, and C. E. Martin: *Sexual Behavior in the Human Male.* Philadelphia: W. B. Saunders, 1948.

Kinsey, A. C., W. B. Pomeroy, E. C. Martin, and P. H. Gebhard: *Sexual Behavior in the Human Female.* Philadelphia: W. B. Saunders, 1953.

McCary, J. L.: *Human Sexuality.* New York: Van Nostrand, 1973.

Madigan, F. C.: "Are Sex Mortality Differentials Biologically Caused," *Milbank Memorial Fund Quarterly,* 1957, **35,** 202–223.

Madigan, F. C., and R. B. Vance: "Differential Sex Mortality: A Research Design," *Social Forces,* 1957, **35,** 193–199.

Masters, W. H., and V. E. Johnson: *Human Sexual Response.* Boston: Little, Brown, 1966.

Masters, W. H., and V. E. Johnson: *Human Sexual Inadequacy.* Boston: Little, Brown, 1970.

Metropolitan Life Insurance Company: "International Trends in Longevity," *Statistical Bulletin,* 1974, **55,** 9–11.

Neugarten, B. L.: "A New Look at Menopause," *Psychology Today,* 1967, **1,** 42–45.

Neugarten, B. L.: "Toward a Psychology of the Life Cycle," in B. L. Neugarten (ed.), *Middle Age and Aging: A Reader in Social Psychology.* Chicago: University of Chicago Press, 1968.

Neugarten, B. L., V. Wood, R. J. Kraines, and B. Loomis: "Women's Attitudes Toward the Menopause," *Vita Humana,* 1963, **6,** 140–151.

Pfeiffer, E., A. Verwoerdt, and H. S. Wang: "Sexual Behavior in

Aged Men and Women," in E. Palmore (ed.), *Normal Aging.* Durham, N.C.: Duke University Press, 1970.

Rose, C. L., and B. Bell: *Predicting Longevity.* Lexington, Mass.: D. C. Heath, 1971.

Ruebsaat, H. J., and R. Hull: *The Male Climacteric.* New York: Hawthorn Books, 1975.

Rutherford, R. D.: "Tobacco Smoking and the Sex Mortality Differential," *Demography,* 1972, **9,** 203–216.

Spiegelman, M.: *Significant Mortality and Morbidity Trends in the U.S. since 1900.* Bryn Mawr, Pa.: American College of Life Underwriters, 1966.

CHAPTER 4

Abbott, M. H., E. A. Murphy, D. R. Bolling, and H. Abbey: "The Familial Component in Longevity: A Study of Offspring of Nonagenarians. II. Preliminary Analysis of the Completed Study," *Johns Hopkins Medical Journal,* 1974, **134,** 1–16.

Beeton, M., and K. Pearson: "Data for the Problem of Evolution in Man. II. A First Study of the Inheritance of Longevity and the Selective Death-Rate in Man, *Proceedings of the Royal Society, London,* 1899, **65,** 290–305.

Bell, A. G.: *The Duration of Life and Conditions Associated with Longevity. A Study of the Hyde Genealogy.* Washington, D.C.: Genealogical Record Office, 1918.

Burks, B. S., D. W. Jensen, L. M. Terman, et al.: "The Promise of Youth: Follow-up Studies of a Thousand Gifted Children," in L. M. Terman (ed.), *Genetic Studies of Genius,* Vol. 3. Stanford, Calif.: Stanford University Press, 1930.

Comfort, A.: *The Biology of Senescence.* New York: Rinehart and Co., 1956.

Comfort, A.: *The Process of Ageing.* New York: New American Library, 1964.

Cox, C. M., L. O. Gillan, et al.: "The Early Mental Traits of Three Hundred Geniuses," in L. M. Terman (ed.), *Genetic Studies of Genius,* Vol. 2. Stanford, Calif.: Stanford University Press, 1926.

Curtis, H. J.: "Biological Mechanisms Underlying the Aging Process," *Science,* 1963, **141,** 686–694.

Cutler, R. G.: "Evolution of Human Longevity and the Genetic Complexity Governing Aging Rate," *Proceedings of the National Academy of Science,* 1975, **72,** 4664–4668.

Goodrick, C. L.: "Life-Span and the Inheritance of Longevity of Inbred Mice," *Journal of Gerontology,* 1975, **30,** 257–263.

Hammond, E. C., L. Garfinkel, and H. Seidman: "Longevity of

Parents and Grandparents in relation to Coronary Heart Disease and Associated Variables," *Circulation*, 1971, **43**, 31–44.

Jalavisto, E.: "Inheritance of Longevity According to Finnish and Swedish Genealogies," *Annals of Medicine International Fenniae*, 1951, **40**, 163–274.

Jarvik, L. F., and J. E. Blum: "Cognitive Declines of Predictors of Mortality in Twin Pairs: A Twenty-Year Longitudinal Study of Aging," in E. Palmore and F. C. Jeffers (eds.), *Prediction of Life Span*. Lexington, Mass.: D. C. Heath, 1971, pp. 199–211.

Jones, K. L., D. W. Smith, M. A. S. Harvey, B. D. Hall, and L. Quan: "Older Paternal Age and Fresh Gene Mutation: Data on Additional Disorders," *Journal of Pediatrics*, 1975, **86**, 84–88.

Kallman, F. J., and G. Sander: "Twin Studies on Senescence," *American Journal of Psychiatry*, 1949, **106**, 29.

Lansing, A. I.: "The Influence of Parental Age on Longevity in Rotifers," *Journal of Gerontology*, 1948, **3**, 6.

Mayo, O., J. L. Murdoch, and T. W. Hancock: "On the Estimation of Parental Age Effects of Mutation," *Annals of Human Genetics*, 1976, **39**, 427–431.

Metropolitan Life Insurance Company: "College Men Long Lived," *Statistical Bulletin*, 1932, **13**, 5–7.

Metropolitan Life Insurance Company: "Longevity of Prominent Men," *Statistical Bulletin*, 1968, **49**, 2–4.

Pearl, R., and R. D. Pearl: *The Ancestry of the Long-Lived*. Baltimore: Johns Hopkins Press, 1934.

Quint, J. V., and B. R. Cody: "Preeminence and Mortality: Longevity of Prominent Men," *American Journal of Public Health*, 1970, **60**, 1118–1124.

Rose, C. L., and B. Bell: *Predicting Longevity*. Lexington, Mass: D. C. Heath, 1971.

Sawin, P. B.: "The Influence of Age of Mother on Pattern of Reproduction," *Annals of the New York Academy of Science*, 1954, **57**, 564–574.

Strehler, B. L.: "Genetic and Cellular Aspects of Life Span Prediction," in E. Palmore and F. C. Jeffers (eds.), *Prediction of the Life Span*. Lexington, Mass.: D. C. Heath, 1971. pp. 33–49.

Terman, L. M., B. T. Baldwin, et al.: "Mental and Physical Traits of a Thousand Gifted Children," in L. M. Terman (ed.), *Genetic Studies of Genius*, Vol. 1 Stanford, Calif.: Stanford University Press, 1925.

Terman, L. M., and M. H. Oden: "The Gifted Child Grows Up: Twenty-five Years' Follow-up of a Superior Group," in L. M. Terman (ed.) *Genetic Studies of Genius*, Vol. 4. Stanford, Calif.: Stanford University Press, 1947.

Terman, L. M., and M. H. Oden: "The Gifted Group at Mid-Life: Thirty-five Years' Follow-up of the Superior Child," in L. M. Terman ed.), *Genetic Studies of Genius*, Vol. 5. Stanford, Calif.: Stanford University Press, 1959.

Wilson, E. B., and C. R. Doering: "The Elder Pierces," *Proceedings of the National Academy of Sciences. United States*, 1926, **12**, 424–432.

Wright, I. S.: "Fulfillment of Hereditary Longevity," *Circulation*, 1976, **54**, 1–2.

Yerushalmy, J.: "Neonatal Mortality by Order of Birth and Age of Parents," *American Journal of Hygene*, 1938, **28**, 244.

Yuan, I.-C.: "Life Tables for a Southern Chinese Family from 1365 to 1849," *Human Biology*, 1931, **3**, 157–179.

CHAPTER 5

Armstrong, B., and R. Doll: "Environmental Factors and Cancer Incidence and Mortality in Different Countries with Special Reference to Dietary Practices," *International Journal of Cancer*, 1975, **15**, 617–631.

Brown, R. C., and L. Ritzmann: "Some Factors Associated with Absence of Coronary Heart Disease in Persons Aged 65 or Older," *Journal of American Geriatrics Society*, 1967, **15**, 239–250.

Butler, R. N.: "Man Does Not Die, He Kills Himself," *International Journal of Aging and Human Development*, 1975, **6**, 367–370.

Connor, W. F., and S .L. Connor: "The Key Role of Nutritional Factors in the Prevention of Coronary Heart Disease," *Preventive Medicine*, 1972, **1**, 49–83.

Denny, P.: "Cellular Biology of Aging," in D. S. Woodruff and J. E. Birren (eds.), *Aging: Scientific Perspectives and Social Issues*. New York: Van Nostrand, 1975, pp. 201–228.

Hakama, M., and E. A. Saxen: "Cereal Consumption and Gastric Cancer," *International Journal of Cancer*, 1967, **2**, 265–268.

Hakulinen T.: "The Increase in Working Years due to Elimination of Cancer as a Cause of Death," *International Journal of Cancer*, 1976, **17**, 429–435.

Hazzard, W. R.: "Aging and Atherosclerosis: Interactions with Diet, Heredity, and Associated Risk Factors," in M. Rockstein and M. L. Sussman (eds.), *Nutrition, Longevity, and Aging*. New York: Academic Press, 1976, pp. 143–195.

Lave, L. B., and E. P. Seskin: "Air Pollution and Human Health," in M. B. Gardner, et al., *Physiological Effects of Air Pollution*. New York: MSS Information Corp. 1973, pp. 184–203.

Lew, E. A.: "High Blood Pressure, Other Risk Factors, and Longevity; The Insurance Viewpoint," *American Journal of Medicine*, 1973, **55**, 281–294.

Peery, T. M.: "The New and Old Diseases: A Study of Mortality Trends in the U.S., 1900–1969," *American Journal of Clinical Pathology*, 1975, **63**, 453–474.

Peery, T. M.: "All-out Effort Cuts Finn's Heart Illness," *The New York Times*, April 3, 1977.

Read, C. R.: "Can We Conquer Cancer?" *Public Affairs Pamphlet* No. 496, 1973.

Read, C. R.: "'76 Cancer Facts and Figures," American Cancer Society, New York, 1975.

Rockstein, M., and M. L. Sussman, (eds.): *Nutrition, Longevity, and Aging*. New York: Academic Press, 1976.

Stamler, J., and F. H. Epstein: "Coronary Heart Disease: Risk Factors as Guides to Preventive Action," *Preventive Medicine*, 1972, **1**, 27–48.

Werko, L.: "Can We Prevent Heart Disease?" *Annals of International Medicine*, 1971, **74**, 278–288.

Whyte, H. M.: "Potential Effect on Coronary-Heart-Disease Morbidity of Lowering the Blood-Cholesterol," *Lancet*, 1975, **1**, 906–910.

CHAPTER 6

Caster, W. O.: "The Role of Nutrition in Human Aging," in M. Rockstein and M. L. Sussman (eds.), *Nutrition, Longevity, and Aging*. New York: Academic Press, 1976, pp. 29–45.

Comfort, A.: *The Process of Ageing*. New York: New American Library, 1964.

Gallup, G., and E. Hill: *The Secrets of Long Life*. New York: Bernard Geis Associates, 1960.

Gerritsen, G. C.: "The Role of Nutrition to Diabetes in Relation to Age," in M. Rockstein and M. L. Sussman (eds.), *Nutrition, Longevity, and Aging*. New York: Academic Press, 1976, pp. 229–252.

Hazzard, W. R.: "Aging and Atherosclerosis: Interactions with Diet, Heredity, and Associated Risk Factors," in M. Rockstein and M. L. Sussman (eds.), *Nutrition, Longevity, and Aging*. New York: Academic Press, 1976, pp. 143–195.

Leaf, A.; "Getting Old," *Scientific American*, 1973, **229**, 44–52.

McCay, C. M., M. F. Crowell, and L. A. Maynard: "The Effect of Retarded Growth upon the Length of Life Span and upon Ultimate Body Size," *Journal of Nutrition*, 1935, **10**, 63–79.

McCay, C. M.: "Chemical Aspects of Ageing and the Effect of Diet upon Ageing," in A. Lansing (ed.), *Cowdry's Problems of Aging.* Baltimore: Williams and Wilkins, 1952, pp. 139–202.

Mickelsen, O.; "The Possible Role of Vitamins in the Aging Process," in M. Rockstein and M. L. Sussman (eds.), *Nutrition, Longevity, and Aging.* New York: Academic Press, 1976, pp. 123–142.

Morrison, L. M.: *The Low-Fat Way to Health and Longer Life.* Englewood Cliffs, N.J.: Prentice-Hall, 1958.

Olefsky, J. M., G. M. Reavan, and J. W. Farquhar: "The Effects of Weight Reduction on Obesity. Studies of Lipid and Carbohydrate Metabolism in Normal and Hyperlipoproteinemic Subjects," *Journal of Clinical Investigation,* 1974, **53**, 64–76.

Ostfeld, A. M.: "Nutritional Aspects of Stroke, Particularly in the Elderly," in M. Rockstein and M. L. Sussman (eds.), *Nutrition, Longevity, and Aging.* New York: Academic Press, 1976, pp. 197–227.

Palmore, E.: "Health Practices, Illness, and Longevity," in E. Palmore and F. C. Jeffers (eds.), *Prediction of Life Span.* Lexington, Mass.: D. C. Heath, 1971, pp. 71–77.

Rockstein, M., and M. L. Sussman (eds.): *Nutrition, Longevity, and Aging.* New York: Academic Press, 1976, see especially "Introduction: Food for Thought," pp. 1–7.

Ross, M. H., and G. Brass: "Food Preference and Length of Life," *Science,* 1975, **190**, 165–167.

Stunkard, A. J.: "Nutrition, Aging, and Obesity," in M. Rockstein and M. L. Sussman (eds.), *Nutrition, Longevity, and Aging.* New York: Academic Press, 1976, pp. 253–284.

Tappel, A. L.: "Where Old Age Begins," *Nutrition Today,* 1967, **2**, 2–7.

CHAPTER 7

Botwinick, J.: *Aging and Behavior.* New York: Springer, 1973.

Field, S. S.: "What Smoking Does to Women," *Reader's Digest,* January 1976, **108**, 94–97.

Gordon, T., W. B. Kannel, and D. McGee: "Death and Coronary Attacks in Men after Giving Up Cigarette Smoking," *Lancet,* 1974, **2**, 1345–1348.

Morrison, L. M.: *The Low-Fat Way to Health and Longer Life.* Englewood Cliffs, N.J.: Prentice-Hall, 1958.

Pearl, R.: "Tobacco Smoking and Longevity," *Science,* 1938, **87**, 216–217.

Peery, T. M.: "The New and Old Diseases: A Study of Mortality Trends in the U.S., 1900–1969," *American Journal of Clinical Pathology,* 1975, **63**, 453–474.

Rogot, E.: "Smoking and Mortality among U.S. Veterans," *Journal of Chronic Diseases*, 1974, **27**, 189–203.

Rogot, E.: *Second-Hand Smoke*. Philadelphia: American Lung Association, 1975.

Rogot, E.: *The Cigarette Controversy*. Washington, D.C.: The Tobacco Institute, 1971.

U.S. Department of Health, Education, and Welfare: *The Surprising News About Women and Smoking*. Washington, D.C.: U.S. Government Printing Office, 1975.

U.S. Public Health Service: *Cigarette Smoking and Health Characteristics*. National Center for Health Statistics, 1967, Series 10, Number 34.

CHAPTER 8

Cahalan, D., I. H. Cisin, and M. Crossley: *A National Study of Drinking Behavior and Attitudes*. New Brunswick, N.J.: Rutgers Center of Alcohol Studies, 1969.

Costello, R. M., and S. L. Schneider: "Mortality in an Alcoholic Cohort," *International Journal of the Addictions*, 1974, **9**, 355–363.

DeLint, J., and T. Levenson: "Mortality Among Patients Treated for Alcoholism: A Five-Year Follow-up," *Canadian Medical Association Journal*, 1975, **113**, 385–387.

Morrison, L. M.: *The Low-Fat Way to Health and Longer Life*. Englewood Cliffs, N.J.: Prentice-Hall, 1958.

Pearl, R.: "Alcohol and Life Duration," *The British Medical Journal*, 1924, **2**, 948–950.

Schmeck, H. M.: "Alcoholism Cost to Nation Put at $25 Billion a Year," *The New York Times*, July 11, 1974.

CHAPTER 9

Adams, G. M., and H. A. deVries: "Physiological Effects of an Exercise Training Regimen upon Women Aged 52 to 79," *Journal of Gerontology*, 1973, **28**, 50–55.

Benet, S.: *Abkhasians: The Long-Living People of the Caucasus*. New York: Holt, Rinehart & Winston, 1974.

Breslow, L., and P. Buell: "Mortality from Coronary Heart Disease and Physical Activity of Work in California," *Journal of Chronic Diseases*, 1960, **11**, 421–444.

Brunner, D., G. Manelis, M. Modan, and S. Levin: "Physical Activity at Work and the Incidence of Myocardial Infarction, Angina Pectoris, and Death due to Ishemic Heart Disease: An Epidemiological Study in Israeli Collective Settlements

(Kibbutzim)," *Journal of Chronic Disease,* 1974, **27,** 217–233.

deVries, H. A.: "Physiological Effects of an Exercise Training Regimen upon Men Age 52 to 88," *Journal of Gerontology,* 1970, **27,** 325–336.

deVries, H. A.: "Prescription of Exercise for Older Men from Telemetered Exercise Heart Rate Data," *Geriatrics,* 1971, **26,** 102–111.

deVries, H. A.: "Exercise Intensity Threshold for Improvement of Cardiovascular-Respiratory Function in Older Men," *Geriatrics,* 1971, **26,** 94–101.

deVries, H. A.: "Physiology of Exercise and Aging," in D. S. Woodruff and J. E. Birren (eds.), *Aging: Scientific Perspectives and Social Issues,* New York: Van Nostrand, 1975, pp. 257–276.

deVries, H. A., and G. M. Adams: "Electromyographic Comparison of Single Doses of Exercise and Meprobamate as to Effects on Muscular Relaxation," *American Journal of Physical Medicine,* 1972, **51,** 130–141.

Drori, D., and Y. Folman: "Environmental Effects on Longevity in the Male Rat: Exercise, Mating, Castration, and Restricted Feeding," *Experimental Gerontology,* 1976, **11,** 25–32.

Frank, C. W., E. Weinblatt, S. Shapiro, and R. B. Sager: "Physical Inactivity as a Lethal Factor in Myocardial Infarction Among Men," *Circulation,* 1966, **34,** 1022–1033.

Gallup, G., and E. Hill: *The Secrets of Long Life,* New York: Bernard Geis Associates, 1960.

Goodrick, C. L.: "The Effects of Exercise on Longevity and Behavior of Hybrid Mice which Differ in Coat Color," *Journal of Gerontology,* 1974, **29,** 129–133.

Goodrick, C. L.: "The Effect of Access to Voluntary Wheel Exercise Throughout the Lifespan upon Longevity of Male and Female Wistar Rats," paper presented at the Annual Meeting of the Gerontological Society, San Francisco, November, 1977.

Hammond, E. C.: "Some Preliminary Findings on Physical Complaints from a Prospective Study of 1,064,004 Men and Women," *American Journal of Public Health,* 1964, **54,** 11–23.

Hammond, E. C., L. Garfinkel, and H. Seidman: "Longevity of Parents and Grandparents in Relation to Coronary Heart Disease and Associated Variables," *Circulation,* 1971, **43,** 31–44.

Kannel, W. B., and I. Gordon (eds): *The Framingham Study: An Epidemiological Investigation of Cardiovascular Disease.* Washington: D.C.: U.S. Government Printing Office, Section 27, December 1970.

Metropolitan Life Insurance Company: "Physical Fitness Test: Seven Years' Experience," *Statistical Bulletin,* 1977, **58,** 2–5.

Morris J. N., J. A. Heady, P. A. B. Raffle, C. G. Roberts, and J. W. Parks: "Coronary Heart Disease and Physical Activity of Work," *Lancet*, 1953, **2**, 1053–1057.

Ready, Set . . . Sweat! *Time*, June 6, 1977, 82–90.

Waters, H. F., L. Whitman, A. R. Martin, and D. Gram: "Keeping Fit: America Tries to Shape Up," *Newsweek*, May 23, 1977, 78–86.

CHAPTER 10

Birren, J. E., and D. S. Woodruff: "A Life-Span Perspective for Education," *New York University Education Quarterly*, 1973, 4, 25–31.

Birren, J. E., and D. S. Woodruff: "Human Development over the Life Span Through Education," in P. B. Baltes and K. W. Schaie (eds.), *Life-Span Developmental Psychology: Personality and Socialization*. New York: Academic Press, 1973, pp. 305–337.

Carnegie Commission on Higher Education: *Less Time, More Options*. New York: McGraw-Hill, 1971.

Eklund, L.: "Aging and the Field of Education," in M. W. Riley, J. W. Riley, Jr., M. E. Johnson, A. Foner, and B. Hess (eds.), *Aging and Society: II. Aging and the Professions*. New York: Russell Sage Foundation, 1969.

Granick, S.: "Cognitive Aspects of Longevity," in E. Palmore and F. C. Jeffers (eds.), *Prediction of Life Span*. Lexington, Mass: D. C. Heath, 1971, pp. 109–122.

Hinkle, L. E., Jr., L. H. Whitney, E. W. Lehman, J. Dunn, B. Benjamin, R. King, A Plakun, and B. Flehinger: "Occupation, Education and Coronary Heart Disease," *Science*, 1968, **161**, 238–246.

Kitagawa, E. M., and P. M. Hauser: *Differential Mortality in the United States: A Study in Socioeconomic Epidemiology*. Cambridge, Mass.: Harvard University Press, 1973.

Metropolitan Life Insurance Company: "College Honor Men Long-Lived," *Statistical Bulletin*, 1932, **13**, 5–7.

Metropolitan Life Insurance Company: "Socioeconomic Mortality Differentials," *Statistical Bulletin*, 1975, **56**, 3–5.

Palmore, E.: "The Relative Importance of Social Factors in Predicting Longevity," in E. Palmore and F. C. Jeffers (eds.), *Prediction of Life Span*. Lexington, Mass.: D. C. Heath, 1971, pp. 237–247.

Pfeiffer, E.: "Physical, Psychological, and Social Correlates of Survival in Old Age," in E. Palmore and F. C. Jeffers (eds.), *Prediction of Life Span*. Lexington, Mass.: D. C. Heath, 1971, pp. 223–236.

Quint, J. V., and B. R. Cody: "Preeminence and Mortality: Longevity of Prominent Men," *American Journal of Public Health*, 1970, **60**, 1118–1124.

Rose, C. L.: "Social Factors in Longevity," *Gerontologist*, 1964, **4**, 27–37.

Rose, C. L., and B. Bell: *Predicting Longevity*. Lexington, Mass.: D. C. Heath, 1971.

Terman, L. M., and M. H. Oden: "The Gifted Group at Mid-Life: Thirty-five Years' Follow-up of the Superior Child," in L. M. Terman (ed.), *Genetic Studies of Genius*, Vol. 5, Stanford, Calif.: Stanford University Press, 1959.

CHAPTER 11

Creagan, E. T., R. N. Hoover, and J. F. Fraumeni: "Mortality from Stomach Cancer in Coal Mining Regions," *Archives of Environmental Health*, 1974, **28**, 28–30.

Dublin, L. I., A. J. Lotka, and M. Spiegelman: *Length of Life: A Study of the Life Table*. New York: Ronald Press, 1949.

Freeman, J. T.: "The Longevity of Gerontologists," *Journal of the American Geriatrics Society*, 1975, **23**, 200–206.

Goodman, L. J..: "The Longevity and Mortality of American Physicians," *The Milbank Memorial Fund Quarterly—Health and Society*, 1975, **53**, 353–375.

Guralnick, L.: "Mortality by Occupation Level and Cause of Death Among Men 20 to 64 Years of Age: United States, 1950. *Vital Statistics—Special Reports, 1963* (National Vital Statistics Division), **53**, 439–612.

Kitagawa, E. M., and P. M. Hauser: *Differential Mortality in the United states: A Study in Socioeconomic Epidemiology*. Cambridge, Mass: Harvard University Press, 1973.

Metropolitan Life Insurance Company: "Longevity of Corporate Executives," *Statistical Bulletin*, 1974, **55**, 2–4.

Metropolitan Life Insurance Company: "Longevity of Presidents of the United States," *Statistical Bulletin*, 1976, **57**, 2–4.

Metropolitan Life Insurance Company: "Recent Trends in Mortality from Accidents," *Statistical Bulletin*, 1976, **57**, 6–19.

Metropolitan Life Insurance Company: "Socioeconomic Mortality Differentials," *Statistical Bulletin*, 1975, **56**, 3–5.

Palmore E.: "The Relative Importance of Social Factors in Predicting Longevity," in E. Palmore and F. C. Jeffers (eds.), *Prediction of Life Span*. Lexington, Mass.: D. C. Heath, 1971, pp. 237–247.

Pearl, R.: *The Rate of Living*. New York: Knopf, 1928.

Powers, E. A., and G. L. Bultena: "Characteristics of Decreased

Dropouts in Longitudinal Research," *Journal of Gerontology,* 1972, **27,** 530–535.

Quint, J. V., and B. R. Cody: "Preeminence and Mortality: Longevity of Prominent Men," *American Journal of Public Health,* 1970, **60,** 1118–1124.

Redmond, C. K., J. Gustin, and E. Kamon: "Long-Term Mortality Experience of Steelworkers," *Journal of Occupational Medicine,* 1975, **17,** 40–43.

Registrar General's Decennial Supplement, England and Wales, 1961. Occupational Mortality Tables, London, HMSO, 1971.

Rose, C. L.: "Social Factors in Longevity," *Gerontologist,* 1964, **4,** 27–37.

Rose, C. L., and B. Bell: *Predicting Longevity.* Lexington, Mass.: D. C. Heath, 1971.

Rowland, K. F.: "Environmental Events Predicting Death for the Elderly," *Psychological Bulletin,* 1977, **84,** 349–372.

Shanas, E.: "Health and Adjustment in Retirement," *Gerontologist,* 1970, **10,** 19–21.

CHAPTER 12

Ayres, S. M., and M. E. Buehler: "The Effects of Urban Air Pollution on Health," *Clinical Pharmacology and Therapeutics,* 1970, **11,** 337–371.

Bogden, J. D.: "Detrimental Health Effects of Noise Pollution," *Journal of the Medical Society of New Jersey,* 1974, **71,** 847–851.

Davis, D. E.: "Physiological Effects of Continued Crowding," in A. Esser (ed.), *Behavior and Environment: The Use of Space by Animals and Man.* New York: Plenum, 1971, pp. 133–147.

Dublin, l. I., A. J. Lotka, and M. Spiegelman: *Length of Life: A Study of the Life Table.* New York: Ronald Press, 1949.

Esser, A. H.: "Experiences of Crowding: Illustration of a Paradigm for Man-Environment Relations," *Representative Research in Social Psychology,* 1973, **4,** 207–218.

Gallup, G., and E. Hill: *The Secrets of Long Life.* New York: Bernard Geis Associates, 1960.

Kramer, M.: "Epidemiology, Biostatistics, and Mental Health Planning," in R. R. Monroe, G. D. Klee, and E. B. Brody (eds.), *Psychiatric Epidemiology in Mental Health Planning. Psychiatric Research Reports of the American Psychiatric Association,* 1967, No. 22, 1–63.

Medvedev, Z. A.: "Caucasus and Altay Longevity: A Biological or Social Problem?" *Gerontologist,* 1974, **14,** 381–387.

Metropolitan Life Insurance Company: "Longevity Patterns in the United States," *Statistical Bulletin*, 1976, **57**, 2–4.

Rose, C. L., and B. Bell: *Predicting Longevity*. Lexington, Mass.: D. C. Heath, 1971.

Sauer, H. I., and D. W. Parke: "Counties with Extreme Death Rates and Associated Factors," *American Journal of Epidemiology*, 1974, **97**, 258–264.

Shepherd, M.: "Pollution, Noise, and Mental Health," *Lancet*, 1975, **1**, 322–333.

Tischler, G. L., J. Henisz, J. K. Myers, and V. Garrison: "Catchmenting and the Use of Mental Health Services," *Archives of General Psychiatry*, 1972, **27**, 385–392.

CHAPTER 13

Aldrich, C. K., and E. Mendkoff: "Relocation of the Aged and Disabled: A Mortality Study," in B. L. Neugarten (ed.), *Middle Age and Aging*. Chicago: University of Chicago Press, 1968, pp. 401–408.

Berkson, J.: "Mortality and Marital Status: Reflections on the Derivation of Etiology from Statistics," *American Journal of Public Health*, 1962, **52**, 1318–1329.

Erikson, E.: *Childhood and Society*, 2nd ed. New York: W. W. Norton, 1963.

Gutman, G. M., and C. P. Herbert: "Mortality Rates Among Relocated Extended-Care Patients," *Journal of Gerontology*, 1976, **31**, 352–357.

Havighurst, R. J.: *Developmental Tasks and Education*, 2nd ed. New York: David McKay, 1972.

Holmes, T. H., and T. S. Holmes: "How Change Can Make Us Ill," in *Stress: A Report from Blue Cross and Blue Shield of Greater New York*, 1974, **25**, 66–75.

Holmes, T. H., and R. H. Rahe: "The Social Readjustment Rating Scale, *Journal of Psychosomatic Research*, 1967, **11**, 213–218.

Kobrin, F., and G. Hendershot: "Mortality: The Life-Giving Properties of Marriage," in J. C. Horn (ed.), *Newsline. Psychology Today*, January 1977, **10**, 20–21.

Komaroff, A. L., M. Masuda, ad T. H. Holmes: "The Social Readjustment Rating Scale: A Comparative Study of Negro, Mexican, and White Americans," *Journal of Psychosomatic Research*, 1968, **12**, 121–128.

Lamott, K.: *Escape from Stress: How to Stop Killing*. New York: G. P. Putnam's, 1974.

Lowenthal, M. F., and C. Haven: "Interaction and Adaptation Intimacy as a Critical Variable," *American Sociological Review*, 1968, **33**, 20–30.

Luce, G. G., and E. Peper: "Learning How to Relax," in *Stress: A Report from Blue Cross and Blue Shield of Greater New York*, 1974, **24**, 84–94.

Ortmeyer, C. E.: "Variations in Mortality, Morbidity, and Health Care by Marital Status," in C. L. Erhardt and J. E. Berlin (eds.), *Mortality and Morbidity in the United States*. Cambridge, Mass.: Harvard University Press, 1974, pp. 159–188.

Pastalan, L., and N. Bourestom: "The Elderly: A Change of Scene Can Be Fatal," in J. C. Horn (ed.), Newsline. *Psychology Today, February* 1977, **10**, 32.

Rahe, R. H., M. Meyer, M. Smith, G. Kjaer, and T. H. Holmes: "Social Stress and Illness Onset," *Journal of Psychosomatic Research*, 1964, **8**, 35–44.

Rowland, K. F.: "Environmental Events Predicting Death for the Elderly," *Psychological Bulletin*, 1977, **84**, 349–372.

Selye, H.: *The Stress of Life*. New York: McGraw-Hill, 1956.

Singer, J. E., and D. C. Glass: "Making Your World More Livable," in *Stress: A Report from Blue Cross and Blue Shield of Greater New York*, 1974, **25**, 59–65.

Toffler, A.: *Future Shock*. New York: Random House, 1970.

U.S. Department of Health, Education, and Welfare: "Differentials in Health Characteristics by Marital Status: United States, 1971–1972," *Vital and Health Statistics* (Data from the National Health Survey), Series 10, No. 104. Washington, D.C.: U.S. Government Printing Office, 1976.

U.S. Department of Health, Education, and Welfare: "Suicides in the United States: 1950–1964," *Vital and Health Statistics* (Data from the National Vital Statistics System) Series 20, No. 5. Washington, D.C.: U.S. Government Printing Office, 1967.

CHAPTER 14

Friedman, M., and R. H. Rosenman: *Type A Behavior and Your Heart*. New York: Fawcett, 1975 (originally published by Alfred A. Knopf, 1974).

Gallup, G., and E. Hill: *The Secrets of Long Life*. New York: Bernard Geis Associates, 1960.

Overholser, R. V., and E. Randolph: "Secrets of How to Live Longer," *Family Circle*, October 1976, **89**, 84–91.

Riegel, K. F., R. M. Riegel, and G. Meyer: "A Study of the Dropout Rates in Longitudinal Research on Aging and the Prediction of Death," in B. L. Neugarten (ed.), *Middle Age and Aging*. Chicago: University of Chicago Press, 1968, pp. 563–570.

Suinn, R. M.: "How to Break the Vicious Cycle of Stress," *Psychology Today*, July 1976, 59–60.

U.S. Department of Health, Education, and Welfare: "Homicide in the United States: 1950–1964," *Vital and Health Statistics* (Data from the National Vital Statistics System) Series 20, No. 6., Washington, D.C.: U.S. Government Printing Office, 1967.

U.S. Department of Health, Education, and Welfare: "Suicides in the United States: 1950–1964," *Vital and Health Statistics* (Data from the National Vital Statistics System) Series 20, No. 5. Washington, D.C.: U.S. Government Printing Office, 1967.

U.S. Department of Health, Education, and Welfare: "Motor Vehicle Accident Deaths in the United States, 1950–1967," *Vital and Health Statistics* (Data from the National Vital Statistics System) Series 20, No. 9. Washington, D.C.: U.S. Government Printing Office, 1970.

U.S. Department of Health, Education, and Welfare: "Mortality Trends for Leading Causes of Death. United States—1950–69," *Vital and Health Statistics* (Data from the National Vital Statistics System) Series 20, No. 16. Washington, D.C.: U.S. Government Printing Office, 1974.

CHAPTER 15

Benet, S.: *Abkhasians: The Long-Living People of the Caucasus,* New York: Holt, Rinehart, and Winston, 1974.

Comfort, A.: *A Good Age.* New York: Crown, 1976.

Cutler, N. E., and R. A. Harootyan: "Demography of the Aged," in D. S. Woodruff and J. E. Birren (eds.), *Aging: Scientific Perspectives and Social Issues.* New York: Van Nostrand, 1975, pp. 31–69.

Leaf, A.: "Getting Old," *Scientific American,* September 1973, **229,** 44–52.

Loeb, M.: "Americans Can—and Should—Live Longer," *Time,* July 10, 1972, **100,** 64–65.

Metropolitan Life Insurance Company: "International Trends in Longevity," *Statistical Bulletin,* October 1974, **55,** 9–11.

Metropolitan Life Insurance Company: "Longevity Patterns in the United States," *Statistical Bulletin,* May 1976, **57,** 2–4.

U.S. Department of Health, Education, and Welfare: "Homicide in the United States: 1950–1964," *Vital and Health Statistics* (Data from the National Vital Statistics System) Series 20, No. 6. Washington, D.C.: U.S. Government Printing Office, 1967.

U.S. Department of Health, Education, and Welfare: "Motor Vehicle Accident Deaths in the United States, 1950–1967," *Vital and Health Statistics* (Data from the National Vital Statistics System) Series 20, No. 9. Washington, D.C.: U.S. Government Printing Office, 1970.

CHAPTER 16

Ettinger, R. C.: *The Prospect of Immortality,* New York: Doubleday, 1964.

Gruman, G. J.: "A History of Ideas About the Prolongation of Life: The Evolution of Prolongevity Hypotheses to 1800," Philadelphia: *Transactions of the American Philosophical Society,* 1966.

Medvedev, Z. A.: "Aging and Longevity: New Approaches and New Perspectives," *Gerontologist,* 1975, **15,** 196–201.

Rosenfeld, A.: *Prolongevity.* New York: Alfred A. Knopf, 1976.

Notes

CHAPTER 2

1. Gruman G. J.: "A History of Ideas about the Prolongation of Life: The Evolution of Prolongevity Hypothesis to 1800," *Transactions of the American Philosophical Society* (Philadelphia, 1966).

CHAPTER 3

1. Rose, C. L., and B. Bell: *Predicting Longevity* (Lexington, Mass.: D. C. Heath, 1971).
2. Benet, S.: *Abkhasians: The Long-living People of the Caucasus* (New York: Holt, Rinehart and Winston, 1974).
3. Comfort, A.: *The Process of Ageing* (New York: New American Library, 1964).
4. Ibid., p. 72.
5. Benet, S.: *Abkhasians.*
6. Neugarten, B. L., V. Wood, R. L. Kraines, and B. Loomis: "Women's Attitudes Toward the Menopause," *Vita Humana,* 1963, **6**, 140–151.
7. Golde, P., and N. Kogan: "A Sentence Completion Procedure for Assessing Attitudes Toward Old People," *Journal of Gerontology,* 1959, **14**, 355–363.
8. Pfeiffer, E., A. Verwoerdt, and H. S. Wang: "Sexual Behavior in Aged Men and Women," in E. Palmore (ed.), *Normal Aging* (Durham, N.C.: Duke University Press, 1970).

CHAPTER 7

1. Morrison, L. M.: *The Low-Fat Way to Health and Longer Life* (Englewood Cliffs, N.J.: Prentice-Hall, 1958) p. 131.
2. Perry, T. M.: "The New and Old Diseases: A Study of Mortality Trends in the U.S., 1900–1969," *American Journal of Clinical Pathology*, 1975, **63**, 465.

CHAPTER 9

1. Gallup, G., and E. Hill: *The Secrets of Long Life* (New York: Bernard Geis Associates, 1969) p. 161.
2. *Ibid.* p. 156.
3. Benet, S.: *Abkhasians: The Long-living People of the Caucasus* (New York: Holt, Rinehart and Winston, 1974) p. 18.

CHAPTER 10

1. Carnegie Commission on Higher Education: *Less Time, More Options* (New York: McGraw-Hill, 1971) p. 2.

CHAPTER 14

1. Gallup, G., and Hill, E.: *The Secrets of Long Life* (New York: Bernard Geis Associates, 1960) pp. 139–140.
2. *Ibid.* pp. 141–142.
3. *Ibid.* p. 145.
4. Friedman, M., and R. H. Rosenman: *Type A Behavior and Your Heart* (New York: Alfred A. Knopf, 1974) pp. 100–102. (Fawcett Edition)
5. *Ibid.* p. 103. (Fawcett Edition)
6. Suinn, R. M.: "How to Break the Vicious Cycle of Stress," *Psychology Today*. July 1976, 59–60.
7. Overholser, R. V., and E. Randolph: "Secrets of How to Live Longer," *Family Circle*, October 1976, **89**, 84–91.
8. *Ibid.*

CHAPTER 16

1. Medvedev, Z. A.: "Aging and Longevity: New Approaches and New Perspectives," *Gerontologist*, 1975, **15**, 196–201.
2. Rosenfeld, A.: *Prolongevity* (New York: Alfred A. Knopf, 1976) p. 166.

About the Author

DIANA S. WOODRUFF, while not herself a centenarian, is a well-known expert on the subject of aging. She has appeared on CBS television in a program dealing with aging and has testified before Congress regarding the Older Americans Act. This book grew out of the public response to her "Longevity Test" which appeared in both *New York* and *New West* magazines. Dr. Woodruff is Associate Professor of Psychology at Temple University and Research Associate of Andrus Gerontology Center at the University of Southern California.

Index